Improving
Access
to

HEALTH
CARE

What Can the States Do?

John H. Goddeeris *and* Andrew J. Hogan
Editors

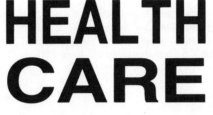

1992

W.E. UPJOHN INSTITUTE for Employment Research
Kalamazoo, Michigan

Library of Congress Cataloging-in-Publication Data

Improving access to health care : what can the states do? / edited by
John H. Goddeeris, Andrew J. Hogan.
    p.   cm.
   Includes bibliographical references and index.
   ISBN 0-88099-117-8 (hard : alk. paper). — ISBN 0-88099-118-6
(pbk. : alk. paper)
   1. Medical policy—United States—States.   2. Right to health
care—United States—States.   I. Goddeeris, John Henry. II. Hogan,
Andrew J.
   [DNLM: 1. Health Policy—United States. 2. Health Services
Accessibility—economics—United States. 3. Insurance, Health—
economics—United States. 4. Medically Uninsured. 5. State
Government. 6. State Health Plans—United States. W 225 I34]
RA395.A3I46 1992
362.1'0973—dc20
DNLM/DLC
for Library of Congress   92–5205
                                                                    CIP

Copyright © 1992
W. E. Upjohn Institute for Employment Research
300 S. Westnedge Avenue
Kalamazoo, Michigan 49007–4686

Cover design by J.R. Underhill
Index prepared by Shirley Kessel
Printed in the United States of America on acid-free paper

ACKNOWLEDGEMENTS

We wish to recognize the contribution of our colleague Steve Woodbury of the Department of Economics at Michigan State University and the W.E. Upjohn Institute for Employment, who conceived of the idea of this volume and who convinced us that editing it would not be half as difficult as it turned out to be. Now that this is over, Steve, we are willing to speak to you again.

Fortunately, we enjoyed excellent support from the Upjohn Institute, from Bob Spiegelman and Allan Hunt. Their belief in this project kept it moving, and they provided us with some insightful editorial commentary of their own. We especially wish to thank Judy Gentry at the Upjohn Institute for her careful and thorough editorial assistance. We thank the other contributors for their patience and persistence in responding to our requests and for producing an excellent set of chapters.

We also recognize the indirect but substantial contributions of the members and staff of the Michigan Governor's Task Force on Access to Health Care, whose insights and commitment to health system reform laid the foundation for this volume. We acknowledge financial support from the Kellogg Foundation and other Michigan foundations for the research underlying many of the chapters. We thank without implicating our colleague Sy Berki of the University of Michigan for his contributions to the work of the Task Force, and for his help in the early stages of this project. To our families and the many others who support us in our lives and work, we thank you for your help in bringing this volume to completion.

John H. Goddeeris
Andrew J. Hogan
East Lansing, MI
February 1992

CONTENTS

Part 1

An Overview of the Access Problem

1
Introduction

John H. Goddeeris
Andrew J. Hogan
Michigan State University

With the 1992 presidential election approaching, deficiencies in the U.S. system of health care finance are beginning to draw national attention. The recent upset election of Harris Wofford (who made support for national health insurance a key plank in his platform) over Richard Thornburgh in Pennsylvania has catapulted health care reform near the top of the political agenda ("Wofford: Costs Are Voters' Key Health Reform Concern" 1991).

A very substantial minority of the population has no insurance coverage of any kind to assist them in buying health care, at a time when one episode of illness requiring hospitalization can easily generate bills in the tens of thousands of dollars. This situation did not suddenly arise in the 1990s. While there has always been at least a significant segment of the population with no health coverage, a combination of trends has begun to bring the problems of access to a head.

- The size of the uninsured population grew substantially in the early 1980s. Although estimates vary on how many are uninsured and how that has changed over time, the number of uninsured under age 65 (almost all of those 65 and over have at least basic coverage through the Medicare program) apparently increased by at least 6 million between 1978 and 1986 (Brown 1989; Congressional Budget Office 1991; see also chapter 2 of this volume).
- The problem of lack of health insurance has been gradually creeping up the income ladder. In the 1970s, the working poor experienced the greatest problems. In the 1980s, the problem was extended to the near poor. A recent study based on the 1991 Current Popula-

tion Survey found that nearly three-fourths of the most recent increase in the uninsured came from families with annual incomes of $25,000 or more (Pear 1991, p. A16).

- Health care costs continue to rise at rates much faster than the general price level or the economy's productive capacity. Cost increases are of great concern in their own right, but they also contribute to fears about access. For one thing, as the cost of health care (and its power to extend life and improve its quality) expands, so may the gap between the standard of care for the well-insured and the uninsured. And as health insurance premiums increase as a share of labor costs, from less than 0.5 percent of total compensation in 1948 to almost 6 percent in 1988 (Piacentini and Cerino 1990, p. 190), many employers who want to provide coverage must seriously consider dropping it, thereby adding to the numbers of the uninsured.
- The old system of implicit subsidies for financing indigent care has eroded. In the past, health care providers could, with relative ease, pass the cost of the care they delivered to the poor uninsured on to the bills paid by the privately insured. But as premium increases mount, employers become far less willing to passively accept this cost shift.

Policymakers in many of the states perceived these trends by the mid-1980s. They were well aware of complaints about the existing financing system from diverse elements of their constituencies: employers, large and small, who were finding it increasingly difficult to maintain coverage for their workers; doctors and hospitals, who felt a moral obligation to provide care but were encountering increasing numbers with no means to pay; and the uninsured and their advocates. But the states also observed a national government that had just slashed income tax rates and was battling large deficits without much success. There appeared to be no federal appetite for considering new social programs or the higher taxes that they might entail.[1]

State policymakers saw no reason to expect prompt action on access to health care at the federal level. A number of states began to look very seriously at the problems of the uninsured to see what they might do on their own. Among them was Michigan, where then-governor James Blanchard convened the Governor's Task Force on Access to Health Care in late 1987. The Task Force was assisted in its deliberations by an Academic Consortium of researchers from the state's major universities. This Consortium was charged with exploring the state's options for expanding access and how much they would cost.

This volume grows out of the Consortium's work. Although the original research was done for the State of Michigan, the authors have tried to distill from what they learned lessons applicable to any state attempting to deal with problems of access. Frequently they use Michigan data for illustrative purposes. While the numbers should be of interest to those in other states, at least as an indication of orders of magnitude, some readers may be more intrigued with the methods of analysis as models that could be applied elsewhere.

In chapter 2, Rashid Bashshur and Cater Webb take a broad look at the problems of access to health care. They provide some background on the U.S. system of health care financing and the increase in the 1980s in the share of the under-65 population with no health coverage. Bashshur and Webb also report data on the makeup of the uninsured population, finding it a diverse group, predominately young and with some connection to the labor force. The employed uninsured, however, tend to work for small firms and to be paid relatively low wages. Bashshur and Webb also note wide variation in the extent of access problems, as measured by lack of coverage, across regions and states. They argue that an important first step for a state attempting to address its problems is to gather data on the nature of its own target population.

Andrew Hogan and John Goddeeris consider in chapter 3 the most radical kind of state response to access problems—the creation of a single-state insurance plan to cover the entire population, perhaps along the lines of those operating in Canadian provinces. Their chapter reviews some of the arguments in favor of a state plan, including those related to more rational delivery of health care from a public health perspective, the potential for administrative savings, and other possible advantages of a single payer for cost control. The authors are, however, skeptical that a politically feasible state plan (see Aaron 1991) would prove effective in controlling cost growth. They emphasize also that a state plan is likely to have substantial redistributional effects as compared with the current system, increasing burdens on the wealthier segments of the population while benefiting the current uninsured or poorly insured poor. Another important issue they identify is the possible loss of significant federal tax subsidies as the financing of health care shifts out of the workplace and onto personal taxes. They illustrate these ideas using data from Michigan.

In chapter 4, Goddeeris looks at another route to universal coverage. The idea is to build on the current employment-based system of health insurance by encouraging employers to cover their workers, and then pick up the remaining uninsured through new public programs. The most likely method for extending employment-based insurance is a "play or pay" tax, whereby employers who do not cover their workers must pay a tax equal to some share of wages. This idea is at the heart of several recent proposals at the national level and has been partially implemented in Massachusetts. Goddeeris discusses a number of issues that arise with this approach. While it might be the most politically feasible route to universal coverage, he argues that it is likely to require more new tax revenue than appears at first glance, as large numbers of individuals who are currently insured find it advantageous to switch to subsidized public coverage. These predictions are borne out in an analysis of Michigan data.

The next chapter considers a more piecemeal approach to dealing with problems of access, one which targets specific populations. One target group includes those small employers who would like to offer insurance but are deterred by costs that are higher for the same coverage than they would be for a larger firm. Hogan and Stephen Woodbury look at the use of pools of small employers, possibly subsidized, as a way of making health insurance more affordable for them. Hogan and Woodbury next consider the implications of making Medicaid available on a buy-in basis for low-income uninsured who do not currently qualify. Another subgroup of the uninsured are those considered uninsurable due to preexisting conditions. Dianne Wolman discusses the experience of a number of states in setting up special pools for these high-risk groups. Finally, if policy initiatives chosen leave some segments of the population uninsured, serious need for care will still exist on the part of individuals with no means to pay. Society may wish to make ar-rangements for financing what would otherwise be uncompensated care. John Herrick and Joseph Papsidero discuss the uncompensated care prob-lem and approaches that various states have taken to dealing with it.

Chapters 6, 7, and 8 deal with more generic issues broadly relevant to policies that attempt to expand access. In chapter 6, David Nerenz and his colleagues discuss the design of benefit packages in health in-surance plans, including considerations of the scope of coverage and the role of cost-sharing. They also discuss how costs of coverage are likely to vary depending on the nature of the benefit package and other factors, and they provide some illustrative calculations based on data from a large Michigan health maintenance organization.

John Anderson takes a public finance perspective in chapter 7. Most public policy initiatives to expand health care access require additional government revenue. Anderson discusses alternative tax instruments, including both increases in rates and expansions of the base for existing taxes, and explores their revenue potential and economic effects. While the amount of revenue needed will influence the choice of instrument, Anderson also emphasizes that it is sound tax policy to look for taxes that distribute the burden fairly and do not unduly distort economic activity.

In chapter 8, Woodbury and Hogan focus on the labor market im-pacts of policies aimed at broadening health care coverage. They offer one of the most comprehensive analyses available of these important issues. The chapter begins with some descriptive analysis of the rela-tionships between health insurance coverage and wage levels, industry of employment, and other factors. The authors go on to analyze the effects of policies like those discussed in chapters 3 through 5, using labor demand and supply analysis. They conclude that for the most part added costs of health insurance, whether imposed on the employer or financed through taxes, will ultimately be borne by the worker in lower after-tax wages (an exception occurs when minimum wage laws pre-vent full backward-shifting of the cost of insurance to workers). A claim is sometimes made that removing health care costs from the workplace, as the creation of a universal tax-financed system could do, would reduce labor costs and thereby improve competitiveness of American business.

Woodbury and Hogan find that unlinking of health insurance from employment is more likely to have the contrary effect of raising labor costs and reducing employment.

Most of the discussion in this volume is in some degree short run, focusing on the needs of the uninsured and the costs of meeting them within a health care delivery system not radically different from what we have. In the final chapter, medical ethicist Leonard Fleck takes a longer view. He argues that deliberations over the future of our health care systems ought to be guided by a well-thought-out vision of what a just society requires. As he points out, asserting that ''health care is a right of all'' does not take us very far, and we as a society must face up to difficult questions of how far that right extends in cases where care is extremely costly and of positive but very limited benefit. Fleck believes that basic moral questions about health care need to be con-fronted and discussed in public forums, in a process that attempts to reach some consensus on how a just society would set limits on access. He describes in some detail a project he has proposed that might serve as one model for such a process of moral conversation and consensus-building.

The Michigan Governor's Task Force issued its report in June 1990. Much of the empirical work on the chapters of this volume was con-ducted around that time. Since then, a major recession has struck Michigan and many other states. State budget deficits have soared, as has the federal budget deficit. Most states are struggling to fund the expansions of the Medicaid program mandated by the federal govern-ment during the late 1980s and have backed away from new initiatives to improve access to health care. The Massachusetts Miracle turned into an economic nightmare, and the new governor has prevented the full implementation of the mandated benefit program passed by the Dukakis administration. In Michigan, tight state finances have led to a backward movement on health care access improvement through the elimination of the General Assistance program. Other states have taken similar measures.

The dire financial predicaments of many of the states have clearly shifted the focus of health care reform back to the federal level. The

Bush administration is being forced, reluctantly, to address the issue. If federal action is not forthcoming as the result of the presidential election, however, and if the economy recovers in 1992, renewed interest at the state level is likely. It is hoped that this volume will assist state policymakers in their deliberations.

NOTE

1. Actually, there was one failed attempt at improving coverage at the federal level. The Medicare Catastrophic Coverage Act expanded Medicare coverage for the elderly through an income-related premium surcharge. The legislation was later repealed due to a groundswell of opposition to the surcharge.

References

Aaron, H.J. 1991. "The Worst Health Care Reform Plan . . . . Except for All the Others," *Challenge* 34(6): 61-63.

Brown, E. Richard. 1989. "Access to Health Insurance in the United States," *Medical Care Review* 46 (Winter): 349-85.

Congressional Budget Office. 1991. *Selected Options for Expanding Health Insurance Coverage* (July).

Pear, R. 1991. "More Are Lacking Health Insurance," *New York Times,* December 19, p. A16.

Piacentini, J.S. and T.J. Cerino. 1990. *EBRI Data Book on Employee Benefits.* Washington, DC: Employee Benefit Research Institute.

"Voters, Sick of Current Health Care System, Want Federal Government to Prescribe Remedy," 1991. *The Wall Street Journal,* June 28, p. A16.

"Wofford: Costs Are Voters' Key Health Reform Concern," 1991. *The Nation's Health* 1(22): 8.

2
Nature and Dimensions of the Problem of Access

Rashid Bashshur
Cater Webb
University of Michigan

Health and Health Care

The principle of health care as a right of citizenship is based on two assumptions: first, that the judicious consumption of health care can and will improve health; and second, that health is necessary to individuals and governments interested in creating and maintaining a free, equal, and productive society. Most countries in the world have explicitly or tacitly endorsed this principle by creating health care systems where no person is denied essential medical services because of inability to pay or other iniquitous reasons.

Despite such efforts, health and universal access to care remain elusive objectives. In their pursuit, all countries attending the World Health Organization's 1978 conference in Alma Ata declared "health for all by the year 2000" as the centerpiece of their national health policies (World Health Organization 1978). The goal of "health for all" encompasses a wide range of specific objectives concerned with health promotion and disease prevention, but it places major emphasis on equity of access to preventive, therapeutic, and rehabilitative health services.

Dimensions of Access

Access to health care is defined as the ability to obtain health services when needed. While major emphasis is often placed on third-party coverage as the determinant of access, the two concepts are not coterminous. Access is assured when the medically insured or financially

11

secure, face no significant barrier to the receipt of care. In that sense, health care coverage is necessary but not sufficient to assure access to health care. Other factors that can act as barriers include the availability of health care facilities or resources within a reasonable distance from where people live, the relative magnitude of opportunity and indirect costs incurred when using health services (such as time and/or wage losses), and the level of human effort involved in the journey for care.[1]

Financial Access

Because they remain formidable, financial barriers to obtaining health care are the most frequently studied in the United States. That is why reference is made to the uninsured when talking about those who lack access to health care. The majority of industrialized nations have more or less successfully addressed financial barriers for their populations by one of three methods: (1) public ownership and public financing of health services, (2) public financing of privately and publicly delivered medical services through universal health insurance programs, or (3) a mix of public and private financing and delivery of care.

The United States falls into the last category, but it is notable for its lack of universal access, although certain public programs have created entitlement for limited segments in the population. For instance, Medicare offers certain health care benefits to nearly all persons over the age of 65; Medicaid covers certain members of the poor, such as families with dependent children, the disabled, blind, the elderly without assets, and occasionally the medically indigent; and the Civilian Health and Medical Program of the Uniformed Services (CHAMPUS) insures the families of military personnel. In addition, the federal government also owns and operates three national health service systems: the Indian Health Service (IHS), the Veterans Administration (VA), and a medical service for all branches of the military. The remaining population does not have entitlement, although the majority are covered by private health insurance plans typically linked with their employment. All told, three out of four Americans had coverage for health care expenses through private health insurance or a mixture of private insurance and public programs in 1987, while another 10 percent had coverage through public programs (Table 1). The remaining 13 to 15 percent of the noninstitutionalized population, numbering approximately 31 to 37 million people, had no health care coverage at all.[2] Thus, the promise "health for all" via universal entitlement to appropriate health services is yet to be fulfilled in the United States.

Table 1
Percentage Distribution of Health Insurance Coverage
of the Civilian Noninstitutionalized Population, by Type of Coverage
United States, 1987

Private Only or Mixture of Private/Public		Public only	Uninsured
Total	**Employment-related**		
74.5	64.3	10.0	15.5

SOURCE: Data computed from Short, Monheit, and Beauregard (1989).

Trends

Certain trends have contributed to growing concern with lack of financial access to health care. Among these are the ever-increasing cost of health services, the growing number of uninsured, and the costs of diminished access for individuals and society.

The Rising Cost of Health Services

The cost of health care as a share of our national income has been increasing rather steadily over the past several decades. The Health Care Financing Administration (HCFA) estimates that national spending on health increased from 5.9 percent of gross national product in 1960 to 11.1 percent in 1988, reaching $539.9 billion in that year (Office of National Health Cost Estimates 1990). If attention is confined to expenditures on personal health care (which excludes government public health spending, spending on medical research, and a few other items), the numbers are somewhat smaller, but the trend is similar (Table 2).

Over the same time period, the proportion of personal health expenditures paid for directly out of consumers' pockets has decreased by about half, from 54.9 percent in 1960 to 27.8 percent in 1987 (Table 3).

Table 2

Growth of Medical Care and Personal Health Care Expenditures and Health Insurance Premiums Expressed as a Ratio of the Average Individual Disposable Income and as a Percentage of the Gross National Product: United States, Selected Calendar Years 1960-1987

Year	Ratio of medical care expenditures to disposable income[a] (%)	Ratio of insurance premiums to disposable income[b] (%)	Personal health care expenditures as a percentage of GNP[c]	National health care expenditures as a percentage of GNP[d]
1960	5.7	2.1	4.6	5.2
1965	6.5	2.5	5.1	5.9
1970	7.7	2.8	6.4	7.4
1975	8.5	3.2	7.3	8.3
1980	9.7	4.4	8.1	9.1
1985	11.4	4.9	9.2	10.3
1986	11.8	4.7	9.5	10.7
1987	n.a.	n.a.	9.7	11.1

SOURCES: Ratios of medical care and insurance premiums to disposable personal income taken from *Source Book of Health Insurance Data: 1988 Update*, Tables 3.1 and 5.10; personal and national health expenditures and GNP are from *Health, United States, 1989*, Tables 100 and 102.

a. Includes all expenses for health care except loss of income.

b. Insurance premiums refers to the combined total of insurance companies' earned premiums, and earned income of Blue Cross-Blue Shield and other hospital-medical plans, as paid for by employers, employees, and persons who purchased individual health insurance plans.

c. Personal health care expenditures are defined as "spending for the direct consumption of health care goods and services" (*Health, United States, 1989*). Since 1950, expenditures for personal health care have totaled between 86 and 89 percent of total expenditures for health care in the United States. As a consequence of using personal health care expenditures, the aggregate ratios of health spending to GNP are lower than those the reader is probably accustomed to.

d. National health expenditures includes expenditures for personal health, program administration, and net cost of private health insurance, government public health activities, and research and construction.

n.a. = not available.

In relative terms, third-party financing—government programs and private insurance—has come to play a much more prominent role in the health sector, although almost all of this expansion occurred prior to 1980. It is interesting to note that out-of-pocket health care expenses as a percentage of disposable income were virtually the same in 1988 as in 1955, at about 3.3 percent (Office of National Health Cost Estimates 1990). Despite the enormous growth of third-party payment over that period, out-of-pocket payments for health care as a share of income did not fall for the average American.

Table 3
Personal Health Care Expenditures in Billions of Dollars and as a Percentage Distribution, by Source of Funds United States, Selected Calendar Years 1960-1987

Year	All sources[a] (100%)	Direct payment (percent)	Private health insurance (percent)	Public payment (percent)
1960	$23.7	54.9	21.1	21.8
1965	35.9	51.6	24.2	22.0
1970	65.4	40.5	23.4	34.3
1975	117.1	32.6	26.7	39.5
1980	219.7	28.7	30.7	39.4
1985	368.3	28.2	30.4	40.2
1986	401.6	28.0	31.0	39.7
1987	442.6	27.8	31.4	39.6

SOURCE: National Center for Health Statistics, *Health, United States, 1989.* Hyattsville, MD: Public Health Service, 1990: 236.
a. Dollar amounts expressed in billions.

Also of interest is the historical trend in the proportion of out-of-pocket costs borne by consumers by type of provider. In 1988, consumers paid 23.7 percent of all expenditures for personal health services, comprising 5.3 percent of hospital care, 18.9 percent of physician services, 48.4 percent of nursing home care, and 51.7 percent of all other expenditures. In 1970, these rates were 39.5 percent overall, comprising 9.0 percent of hospital care, 42.8 percent of physician services, 48.2 percent of nursing home care, and 80.6 percent of all other expenditures (Table 4).

Table 4
Percentage of Consumer Expenditures Paid Out-of-Pocket
for Selected Health Care Providers
United States, Selected Calendar Years 1960-1988

	1960	1970	1980	1988
		(percent)		
Total	55.9	39.5	26.8	23.7
Hospital care	20.7	9.0	5.2	5.3
Physician care	62.7	42.8	26.9	18.9
Nursing home care	80.5	48.2	43.3	48.4
All other	87.5	80.6	61.4	51.7

SOURCE: Abstracted from Office of National Health Cost Estimates (1990).

It should be emphasized that out-of-pocket expenses do not measure the full burden of health care costs on individuals. Leaving aside the taxes needed to finance public coverage, out-of-pocket payments do not include health insurance premiums, which are a burden on individuals either directly or as a substitute for other forms of employee compensation. If we simply add payments for health insurance to out-of-pocket costs, the total amounts to 48 percent of all personal health care expenditures (Short 1988).

Lack of Third-Party Coverage

Given the high cost of health care, lack of coverage through a public program or private insurer presents a formidable financial barrier to obtaining medical services for many Americans. During the 1980s, individuals without any third-party health care coverage increased both in absolute numbers and as a percentage of the civilian noninstitutionalized population. Approximately 18 million individuals, corresponding to 9.5 percent of the U.S. population, were uninsured in 1977, whereas this estimate had risen to about 37 million individuals or 15.5 percent of the population, a decade later.[3] Preliminary results from the March

1988 and 1989 Current Population Survey (CPS) suggest a decline in the proportion and number of the uninsured to 31 million or 13 percent in 1988, and 33 million or 15 percent in 1989. However, the change may simply reflect a methodological artifact resulting from changes in the survey instrument and coding procedures.[4]

Private Coverage: The decline in health care coverage has occurred in both private and public sectors, but for different reasons. The decline of health insurance in the private sector can generally be attributed to the linking of insurance coverage and employment. By coupling health insurance to employment, health care coverage is subject to the vagaries of the marketplace, and it flows and ebbs with the fluctuations in the business cycle and changes in occupational and employment patterns.

One of the serious consequences of employer-linked insurance coverage that does not receive adequate attention is temporary loss of insurance, referred to as "uninsured spells" (Swartz and McBride 1990). Swartz and McBride estimated that "half of all uninsured spells end within four months while only 15 percent last longer than 24 months." Recent analysis of census data has revealed that 63 million Americans were uninsured for at least one month during a 28-month period in 1985-1987 (Short 1988).

In a cohort study of privately insured and uninsured persons over a 32-month period, Monheit and Schur (1988) found substantial "volatility in health insurance status," especially among the uninsured. They concluded that the "uninsured population is quite heterogeneous," consisting of individuals who lose coverage for relatively short periods of time, individuals without insurance for extended periods of time, and individuals who are regularly uninsured. This is so despite the fact of COBRA (Consolidated Omnibus Budget Reconciliation Act of 1985), which mandated firms with 20 or more workers to offer employees who become ineligible for health benefits the opportunity to continue group insurance benefits for themselves and their dependents. Firms are allowed to charge employees up to 102 percent of the premiums. If the newly ineligible employees can pay the premiums, coverage can be continued for up to 18 months if they no longer work for the firm or if their hours have been reduced. Coverage is extended to 36 months when ineligibility is due to divorce, legal separation, Medicare entitlement, or a dependent child's passing the age where coverage is terminated by the plan (U.S. General Accounting Office 1989, p. 50). The difficulty of making the premium payments has apparently limited the number of eligibles who take advantage of the COBRA provisions.

A more specific result of the employment-health insurance linkage is suggested by Renner and Navarro (1989), who argue that the "deindustrialization" of America has been the major cause of the decline in private insurance in the United States. While there is debate over what constitutes deindustrialization (Kutscher and Personick 1986), generally the term refers to the movement from a manufacturing-based economy to a service-based economy. Although the goods-producing sector (the manufacturing, construction, mining, and agricultural industries) has maintained a large share of its labor force overall, employment growth during the past few decades has been almost exclusively in service-producing industries, whose share of the economy's jobs almost doubled between 1960 and 1989 (Table 5). The growth of the service industry has paralleled a relative decline in the manufacturing industries, with the share of manufacturing jobs decreasing by almost one-third from 1960 to 1989. It has been projected that by 1995, four out of five new (nonagricultural) jobs will be in the service sector (Personick 1987).

One aspect of these changes in the labor market is "worker displacement." Displaced workers are individuals who, through no fault of their own, have lost jobs in which they had made substantial investment in time and training, usually three or more years. In a supplement to the January 1988 Current Population Survey, designed to study displacement, it was found that workers in goods-producing industries were two to six times more likely to be displaced than workers in service industries from 1983 to 1987, even though this was a period of rapid job expansion. Furthermore, three out of every four workers displaced during this period reported having had some type of health insurance coverage when employed at their lost jobs, but half of those still unemployed at the time of the survey were without insurance; four out of ten who had dropped out of the workforce no longer had group health coverage; and 20 percent of the reemployed were still without insurance (Herz 1990).

Table 5
Percentage Distribution of Nonagricultural Employment
in the Manufacturing and Service Industries, and
Probability of Being Uninsured by Industry
United States, Selected Calendar Years 1960-1987

Combined industrial categories	1960	1979	1987	1989	Probability of being uninsured (1987)
		(percent)			(percent)
Manufacturing[a]	31.0	23.5	18.6	18.1	10.2
Services[b]	13.6	18.7	23.6	24.8	13.3

SOURCES: Data for industry percentage distributions in 1960 and 1987 taken from U.S. Bureau of Labor Statistics as published in U.S. Bureau of the Census (1989, p. 397). Data for 1979 tabulated from Table 6 in V. Personick (1987). Data for 1989 based on average of seasonally adjusted quarterly averages in Table 1 in S.E. Haugen and W. Parks, "Job Growth Moderated in 1989 While Unemployment Held Steady," *Monthly Labor Review* (February 1990) 3-16. Probabilities of being uninsured by industry based on Government Accounting Office tabulations of 1987 CPS data reported in U.S. General Accounting Office (1990).
a. The manufacturing industry includes durable and nondurable goods.
b. The services industry includes business and repair, personal, entertainment and recreation, and professional services.

More specifically, deindustrialization is associated with three changes in the composition of the labor force, all of which have negatively affected private insurance coverage for workers and their dependents (Renner and Navarro 1989, pp. 86-90). Employment patterns have shifted from union to nonunion labor, from full-time to part-time work loads, and from high-paying manufacturing jobs to low-paying service jobs, all contributing to a decrease in employer-provided health insurance benefits for workers. Unions played a major role in securing health insurance coverage in the standard wage-compensation package in the Northeast and North Central regions of the United States after World War II (Swartz 1989, p. 2), and they continue to play a key role in maintaining health insurance benefits (Ruben 1990). The percentage of the entire labor force with union membership has receded from 35 percent in 1954 to 16.1 percent in 1985 (Doyle 1985).

When measured in current dollars, the 1970 average weekly earnings in manufacturing were 37 percent higher than in services, and 47 percent higher by 1987.[5] At least part of the growth in service industries has been in part-time jobs, with average weekly hours dropping from 35.9 to 32.5 from 1960 to 1987.[6] Another measure of the shift to services is that share of worker hours dropped in the goods-producing sector from 41.1 percent in 1959 to 30.3 percent in 1984 (Kutscher and Personick 1986, p. 7). Among service workers, average weekly earnings (as measured in constant 1977 dollars) dropped from $151 in 1970 to a low of $140 in 1980, then rose slowly to $149 by 1987, which is still below 1970 levels. In the same time period, the average weekly earnings for the manufacturing industries rose steadily from $208 to $220.

Hence, the basic problem is that overall real wages declined during the 1970s, and they have not yet rebounded fully. At the same time, health care costs in real dollars kept increasing, with more people being priced out.

Public Coverage: The decline in the proportion of people covered by public programs, particularly Medicaid, can be attributed in large part to the tightening of the categoric eligibility requirements for benefits as a consequence of the Omnibus Budget Reconciliation Act of 1981 (OBRA). OBRA was designed to reduce spending, and it was successful in curbing the rate of increase in expenditures by reducing the size of the federal matching funds to state expenditures, restricting eligibility for welfare benefits such as Medicaid, and permitting states to change reimbursement and administrative systems, including the change from a retrospective cost-based hospital reimbursement system, which is generally held to increase costs, to a prospective payment system.[7] The tightening of eligibility requirements reduced access for the working poor, who constitute approximately two-thirds of the uninsured (Employee Benefit Research Institute 1990, p. 1).

The Medicaid Program Evaluation, published in 1987, reported that the annual rate of increase in Medicaid expenditures dropped by about one-half during the period from 1981 to 1984, and that reductions in expenditures per Medicaid recipient accounted for 85 percent of the total decrease in growth. Declines in spending affected adults and children, while expenditures per recipient increased 2 to 3 percent for the aged, blind, and disabled. Slowed growth in spending occurred despite the fact that the number of persons whose income was below the federal poverty line increased by 10 million between 1979 and 1983, and that the sharpest increase occurred in the number of families with incomes below 50 percent of poverty, up 66 percent.

The Costs of Diminished Access to Health Care

A theoretically optimal system of care to achieve "health for all" with the proper levers for an effective control of use of service would necessarily encourage appropriate use of care (i.e., assure access for people who have legitimate need for care), while discouraging care when not medically indicated. In such a system, access to care would be assured at a level that is no more and no less than is necessary to restore, sustain, or promote health, or else to ameliorate pain and suffering when all else fails. The design of such a system has been elusive, however, and we are mired in a system of unbalanced incentives and controls. The primary utilization controls that have been imposed on patients are based on the assumption that increasing their direct costs may prompt them to become smarter consumers of health care and use the proper mix of services. Yet, evidence from the Rand Health Insurance Experiment suggests that the average person is unable to differentiate between what is necessary or appropriate and what is not, and that once the decision to see the physician is made, it is the doctor and not the patient who chooses the service mix.[8]

When requiring expensive medical treatment, the uninsured and those with inadequate coverage find themselves in a real predicament: to forgo the needed care; to lose their savings and their assets (if any) to obtain it; or else to renege on paying, thereby shifting the burden to the provider. There is evidence that all three options occur in varying degrees.

Data from a 1986 survey supported by the Robert Wood Johnson Foundation revealed that approximately one million Americans could not obtain health care that year because they could not afford it. Another 19 million reported that they required services but faced financial barriers in obtaining them.[9] The survey also found that, compared to people who had health insurance, the uninsured were somewhat less likely to obtain preventive services such as immunizations for young children (94 percent versus 81 percent) and prenatal care in the first trimester (85 percent versus 80 percent). They were also 13 percent less likely to see a physician in a 12-month period, overall. In addition, the uninsured were 48 percent less likely than the insured to see a physician within 30 days for serious symptoms such as persistent high fever, nausea, or bleeding (Brown 1989). A study compared the utilization behavior of three types of Medicare recipients: (1) those who had Medicare only; (2) those with Medicare and Medicaid (about 13 percent of the noninstitutionalized elderly); and (3) those with Medicare and private medigap-types of insurance. The researchers found that the number of outpatient visits was lower for those who had only Medicare, as compared to those who had Medicare and medigap, while the highest outpatient visit rates were observed among those with both Medicare and Medicaid. In terms of hospitalization, private supplemental insurance increased the likelihood of admission. However, no differences among the three types of coverage were found with regards to length of stay, including the small proportion of those without any coverage (Dunlop, Wells, and Wilensky 1989).

While forgoing unnecessary care for minor or self-limiting conditions may have neutral, or possibly positive, effects on health, unattended illness may lead to further deterioration in health, often requiring subsequently more expensive treatment. This is ironic because preventive care is not only relatively inexpensive, it may also lead to long-term savings by enabling early detection and less costly treatment of certain diseases. For example, a study by the General Accounting Office (GAO) found that Medicaid recipients and uninsured women began prenatal care later than did privately insured women, and they had fewer visits, overall (U.S. General Accounting Office 1988). Women with inadequate prenatal care were more likely to have low birth weight babies, and such babies cost between $14,000 and $30,000 in hospitalization during the first year and in long-term health care costs. "For every $1 spent for prenatal care for high-risk women, an estimated $3.38 can be saved by preventing costs associated with low birth weight."[10]

When the uninsured receive services, they may be unable to pay for them, thereby resulting in uncompensated care which includes both bad debt and charity or free care. We do not have reliable estimates of un-compensated care provided by physicians. However, estimates for hospitals indicate a growing problem. For instance, it is estimated that uncompensated hospital costs jumped from $2.8 billion to $7.2 billion between 1980 and 1987. This increase occurred while changes in reim-bursement made cross-subsidization of such financial burdens more dif-ficult (King 1989, p. 32).

Profile of the Uninsured

In this part of the chapter, we describe the characteristics of the un-insured and those on public programs in the United States, and their variations by region and state. The inclusion of data on public coverage is predicated on (1) the observed association between the decrease in the number of individuals covered by Medicaid and the increase in the number of uninsured, and (2) the assumption that Medicaid is the most feasible mechanism available to the states for expanding health care coverage for the uninsured within the existing system. Hence, by know-ing the levels of Medicaid coverage in each state, the potential for fur-ther expansion of Medicaid can be assessed. For instance, states with a high uninsured rate and a low rate of Medicaid coverage may be more able to expand Medicaid coverage than states already encumbered with high rates of Medicaid coverage, other things being equal. In addition to these data, we present a special analysis of health care coverage in Michigan from a 1989 survey as an example of the type of information necessary for developing policy at the state level.

Persons lacking coverage in the United States will be described in terms of socio-demographic, economic, and employment characteristics (data shown in Table 6, Table 7, and Table 8). These variables are im-portant for policy formulation because they identify who the uninsured are in terms of significant social and economic variables that can serve as the basis for possible solutions. For example, the size of the uninsured

Table 6
Size and Distribution of the Civilian Noninstitutionalized Population, by Type of Health Care Coverage and Selected Population Characteristics: United States, 1987

Population characteristic	Number in thousands	Total population (percentage)	Private third-party coverage (percentage)	Public coverage only (percentage)	Uninsured
Total	237,890	100.0	74.5	10.0	15.5
Age					
18 and younger	67,106	28.2	26.7	35.8	30.7
19-24	22,675	9.5	8.1	6.2	18.7
25-64	120,200	50.6	53.4	29.5	49.9
65 and older	27,909	11.7	11.8	28.5	0.7
Sex					
Male	115,148	48.4	48.8	40.0	52.1
Female	122,743	51.6	51.2	60.0	47.9
Marital status					
Married	105,024	44.2[a]	49.5[a]	24.2[a]	31.4[a]
Single	40,532	17.0	15.1	14.4	28.0
Divorced & separated	18,556	7.8	6.4	12.8	11.1
Widowed	13,551	5.7	5.1	15.2	2.4
Ethnicity					
White	182,794	76.8[b]	83.3[b]	52.0[b]	61.7[b]
Black	28,356	11.9	8.5	29.8	17.0
Hispanic	18,752	7.9	5.3	14.4	16.1

SOURCE: Data computed from Short, Monheit, and Beauregard (1989).
a. Figures add to less than 100 percent because marital status of persons under age 17 was not ascertained.
b. Figures add to less than 100 percent because of missing data.

Table 7

Probabilities and Percentage Distributions of Individuals With Public Coverage Only or No Insurance, by Selected Socio-Demographic and Economic Characteristics: United States, 1987

Population characteristic	Probability of		Percentage distribution[a]	
	Public coverage only (%)	Uninsured (%)	Public coverage only	Uninsured
Total	10.0	15.5	100.0	100.0
Age				
18 and younger	12.7	16.8	35.8	30.7
19-24	6.5	30.2	6.2	18.7
25-64	5.9	15.3	29.5	49.9
65 and older	24.4	0.9	28.5	0.7
Sex				
Male	8.3	16.6	40.0	52.1
Female	11.7	14.3	60.0	47.9
Marital status				
Married	5.5	11.0	24.2	31.4
Single	8.5	25.4	14.4	28.0
Divorced & separated	16.3	22.0	12.8	11.1
Widowed	26.6	6.6	15.2	2.4
Ethnicity				
White	6.8	12.4	52.0	61.7
Black	25.1	22.0	29.8	17.0
Hispanic	18.3	31.5	14.4	16.1

SOURCE: Data computed from Short, Monheit, and Beauregard (1989).
a. Due to missing data, the percentage distribution figures may not add to 100 percent.

Table 8
Population Size, Probability and Percentage Distributions of the Uninsured, by Type of Family and Employment Status of Family Head: United States, 1987

Family characteristic	Number of uninsured (millions)	United States Probability of being uninsured (%)	Percentage of uninsured	Michigan[b] Probability of being uninsured (%)	Percentage of uninsured
Total families, by type:[a]	31.1	12.9	100.0	10.1	100.0
Single with dependents	5.1	19.2	16.4	11.8	17.1
Couple with dependents	11.2	11.0	36.1	8.9	40.0
Single, no dependents	8.9	18.9	28.6	18.3	36.6
Two or more adults, no dependents	5.9	9.0	18.9	3.3	6.3
Uninsured families by employment status of adults in family:[c]					
Total	36.8	15.5	100.0	n.a.	n.a.
Total in families with a working adult:	28.2	15.2	76.6	n.a.	n.a.
Working adult	17.1	15.2	46.5	n.a.	n.a.
Nonworking spouse	2.5	15.6	6.8	n.a.	n.a.
Child of working adult	8.6	15.1	23.3	n.a.	n.a.
Total in families without a working adult:	5.9	8.6	16.4	23.4	n.a.
Nonworking adults	2.7	11.3	16.0	n.a.	n.a.
Children		5.1	7.4	n.a.	n.a.

SOURCES: Computed from Exhibit 2 in Moyer (1989); Table 2 in Short, Monheit, and Beauregard (1989); and Bashshur et al. (1989).
a. Preliminary tabulations from the March 1988 Current Population Survey.
b. Calculated from 1989 HISM data.
c. Tabulations from the 1987 National Medical Expenditure Survey-Household Survey, Round 1.
n.a. = Not ascertained due to small number of cases in the sample.

population reveals the magnitude of the problem, be it at the state or national level. Age, sex, and dependency status provide important clues regarding the nature of need in the target populations; employment attributes and income levels might suggest the potential for securing coverage through employment, be it subscriber- or employer-paid.

Socio-Demographic Characteristics

Approximately 14 to 17 percent, or 33 to 37 million Americans are uninsured (EBRI 1990; Short 1988, p. 4). Half of the uninsured are between 25 and 65 years of age, another 30 percent, or 11.1 million, are children 18 years of age or younger, and the remaining 20 percent are between 19 and 25 (Table 7). Less than 1 percent of the uninsured are over 65. The largest proportion of persons with public coverage only are children less than 18 (35.8 percent), followed by adults between 25 and 64 years of age, adults 65 years of age and older, and young adults age 19 to 25.

There are slightly more males than females among those without any third-party coverage, but three out of five of those covered by public programs only are female.

Thirty percent of the uninsured are married, 28 percent single, 11 percent divorced or separated, and only 2.4 percent are widowed. The distribution for public coverage only is slightly different. A quarter are married, but the next largest group is the widowed at 15 percent, followed by single individuals, and finally the divorced and separated.

Nearly two-thirds of the uninsured are white, 17 percent are black, 16 percent are Hispanic, and the remaining 5 percent are other minorities. The same overall trends are seen for public coverage. Over half of the individuals with public coverage are white, about 30 percent are black, 14 percent are Hispanic, and 3.8 percent are other minorities.

The vulnerability of the American family to lack of financial access to health care, through private health insurance or public coverage, is revealed in the data provided in Table 8. More than one-third of all the uninsured are couples with dependent children; another 16.4 percent are single parents with dependent children. Together, single-parent and two-parent families constitute 52.5 percent of the uninsured in the country.

Economic and Employment Characteristics

While the data on the socio-demographic characteristics of the un-insured and public program participants help identify the target population, information on employment characteristics and income is necessary for designing programs to assist the uninsured. This is particularly important if the new coverage is connected to employment, through either voluntary or mandatory means.

The economic and employment profile of the uninsured is presented in terms of employment status, size of firm, type of industry, union affiliation, employment status of adults in the family, family income, and ratio of family income to poverty. These data are for persons below age 65, with children classified according to the characteristics of the head of household. Data are presented in Tables 8, 9 and 10.

Although the uninsured population includes individuals of widely varying characteristics, most prominently the uninsured are full-time workers in relatively small firms in the service sector. They are usually not members of unions, and most commonly earn less than $10 per hour.

About 77 percent of the uninsured are in families with at least one working adult (Table 8). From a policy perspective, this suggests that coverage extended through the workplace (for dependents and other family members) can reach three-quarters of the uninsured, provided such action did not reduce employment. Of the employed uninsured, the majority, or 61 percent, ar working on a full-time basis; another 19 percent are working part time, and 19 percent are self-employed. Considering only the uninsured employed and their dependents, 61 percent are working adults, 9 percent are nonworking spouses, and 30 percent are children. The remainder of the uninsured live in families without a working adult, and among the nonworking uninsured, one-third are children.

In terms of firm size, one-third of the employed uninsured are in small firms with fewer than 10 workers, 25 percent are employed by medium-sized firms with between 10 and 100 workers, and 10.7 percent are in large firms with over 100 workers (Table 9).

One in five of the uninsured is engaged in sales, and another 22 percent are in other service industries, which include repair, personal and

Table 9
Probabilities and Percentage Distributions of Uninsured Individuals Under 65 Years of Age by Employment Characteristics:[a]
United States, 1987

Employment characteristic	Number of uninsured (millions)[b]	Probability of being uninsured (%)	Percentage distribution of uninsured[b]
Total	37.0	15.6	100.0
Employment status			
Full time	17.1	12.7	46.2
Part time	5.4	24.1	14.7
Self-employed	5.4	22.9	14.7
Unemployed/not in		42.0[c]	
the labor force	9.1[c]	18.0[c]	24.4[c]
Size of firm			
Less than 10 workers	12.5	26.3	33.7
10 - 25 workers	4.9	17.8	13.3
26 - 100 workers	4.3	12.3	11.7
Over 100 workers	2.0	6.0	5.3
Industry			
Agriculture	1.4	29.6	3.8
Mining	0.2	10.0*	0.5*
Construction	3.9	30.6	10.6
Manufacturing	3.8	10.3	10.3
Transportation &			
communications	1.6	10.4	4.3
Sales	6.8	21.4	18.3
Financial services	1.3	8.3	3.5
Repair services	2.3	21.6	6.2
Personal services	1.7	31.5	4.7
Professional services	3.6	10.5	9.8
Entertainment	0.6	30.2	1.5
Public administration	0.8	7.1	2.2
Union affiliation			
Member	0.9	5.2	2.4
All others	27.0	16.5	72.9

SOURCES: Table 6 in Short, Monheit, and Beauregard (1989), p. 11; and Tables 7 and 8 in U.S. General Accounting Office (1990, p. 9).

a. Computed from 1987 NMES data. Working adults classified according to their own employment characteristics. Nonworking spouses and children are classified according to the characteristics of the worker. Children of two working parents are classified according to the characteristics of the male head of household. Figures also include individuals with unknown employment status, establishment size, union membership or wages.

b. Due to missing data, the population figures and percentage distributions of the uninsured within characteristics may not add to the totals.

c. From GAO tabulations of March 1987 CPS data. Separate estimates of the probability of having no insurance were made for unemployed and those not in the labor force, however, the two categories were combined in the report of the distribution of the uninsured by employment status.

*Relative standard error is greater than or equal to 30 percent.

professional services, and entertainment. A quarter of the uninsured work in the production sector, with the majority in construction or mining, which have about 10 percent each.

The distribution of the uninsured by hourly wage shows that most of those working earn between $3.50 and $10 per hour (Table 10). About one in three of the uninsured have family incomes below $10,000 a year, and another third have annual incomes between $10,000 and $20,000. At the other end of the spectrum, about 22 percent, or one in five, of the uninsured have family incomes above $30,000 a year. The distribution of the uninsured with respect to poverty (a measure that adjusts family income to family size) is quite similar, with about a third whose annual incomes are at or below the federal poverty line, 30 percent with incomes between 100 and 200 percent of poverty, and 37 percent with incomes exceeding 200 percent of poverty. It should be noted that 33 percent of this last group have incomes between 200 and 500 percent of poverty; 9 percent of the uninsured have incomes that are five or more times larger than a poverty income.[11]

Variation by Region and State

The variations in the distribution and absolute numbers of the uninsured between regions are quite substantial (Table 11). Census data for 1986 revealed that 15.3 million, or 41.3 percent, of the uninsured lived in the South, followed by the West with 8.6 million, or 23.3 percent. Approximately 7.2 million, or 19.5 percent, of the uninsured lived in the Midwest, while 5.9 million, or 15.9 percent, lived in the Northeast.

Disparity between the states is quite obvious. In order to give complete information on this question, we grouped the states into three strata: (1) states with low levels of insurance coverage, defined as having 20 percent or more uninsured; (2) states with a medium level of insurance, defined as having between 15 and 20 percent uninsured; and (3) states with high levels, defined as having under 15 percent uninsured. The data are shown in Table 12.

Table 10
Nonelderly Uninsured Population, by Income, Poverty,
and Hourly Wages: United States, 1987

Income	Probability of being uninsured (%)	Percentage distribution of uninsured[a]
Total	15.6	100.0
Hourly wage		
$3.50 or less	30.1	7.6
$3.51-$5.00	30.4	19.7
$5.01-$10.00	14.6	24.4
$10.01-$15.00	6.6	6.5
Over $15.00	5.1	3.7
Family income[b]		
Under $5,000	35.4	14.3
$5,000-$9,999	33.9	16.1
$10,000-$14,999	33.3	17.2
$15,000-$19,999	25.8	13.5
$20,000-$29,999	15.6	16.6
$30,000-$39,999	9.3	9.2
$40,000 or more	5.5	13.1
Ratio of family income to poverty		
In poverty	37.1	33.0
100-199 percent	29.2	30.0
200 percent or more	9.0	37.0

SOURCES: Family income data from Employment Benefit Research Institute tabulations of the March 1989 CPS, corrected Table 3 in EBRI (1990), 104, p. 7. Poverty data from U.S. General Accounting Office tabulations of March 1987 CPS data, Tables 4 and 5 in U.S. General Accounting Office (1990, p. 8). Hourly wage data from Short, Monheit, and Beauregard (1989), p. 11.
a. Due to missing data, the percentage distributions of the uninsured may not add to 100 percent.
b. 1988 data.

Table 11
Population Size, Percentage Distribution, Probability of Being Uninsured, and the Probability
of Having Public Coverage Only, for Persons Under 65 Years of Age,
by Geographic Region: United States, 1986

Region	Population in millions	Percentage distribution of uninsured	Probability of being uninsured (%)	Probability of having only public coverage (%)
Total	37.0	100.0	16.3	10.0
Census region				
Northeast	5.9	15.9	11.3	10.3
Midwest	7.2	19.5	11.2	9.2
South	15.3	41.3	18.9	11.4
West	8.6	23.3	19.3	8.5
More detailed regions				
Northeast				
New England	1.3	3.5	12.2	9.1
Middle Atlantic	4.6	12.4	14.3	11.5
Midwest				
East-North Central	5.1	13.8	14.1	12.3
West-North Central	2.1	5.7	14.0	10.2
South				
South Atlantic	6.4	17.3	18.5	11.2
East-South Central	3.0	8.0	22.7	13.9
West-South Central	5.9	16.0	25.2	11.4
West				
Mountain	2.2	6.0	19.7	9.6
Pacific	6.4	17.3	20.5	13.6

SOURCE: Data computed from the Employment Benefit Research Institute tabulations of the March 1987 Current Population Survey, in Source Book of Health Insurance Data, 1989.

Table 12
Population Size, Percentage Distribution of Persons Under 65 Years of Age With No Insurance and Public Coverage Only, and the Ratio of the Uninsured to Public Coverage Populations, for Individual States Arranged by Their Level of Private Health Insurance Coverage: United States, 1986

States by level of private insurance	Total population (000)	Percentage with public coverage only	Percentage uninsured	Uninsured to public coverage (%)
Low level				
Mississippi	2,249	13.5	27.0	200
Texas	14,569	9.8	26.3	268
New Mexico	1,249	11.4	26.0	228
Arkansas	2,007	14.7	24.3	165
Alabama	3,575	12.0	24.0	200
Florida	9,653	10.4	23.2	223
Louisiana	3,920	15.3	23.1	151
Oklahoma	2,793	11.9	22.8	192
Idaho	863	n.a.	22.7	n.a.
Arizona	2,895	7.6	22.5	296
California	23,874	13.7	21.5	157
Alaska	453	n.a.	21.4	n.a.
District of Columbia	526	n.a.	21.3	n.a.
Kentucky	3,139	14.3	21.0	147
Tennessee	4,010	15.5	21.0	135
Mid-level				
Oregon	2,401	9.7	19.9	205
Montana	715	12.3	18.7	152

Table 12 (continued)

States by level of private insurance	Total population (000)	Percentage with public coverage only	Percentage uninsured	Uninsured to public coverage (%)
North Carolina	5,364	9.9	18.4	186
West Virginia	1,621	18.3	18.2	99
Georgia	5,311	12.7	18.0	142
Delaware	553	n.a.	17.9	n.a.
Indiana	4,654	7.3	17.9	245
Wyoming	441	n.a.	17.7	n.a.
Nevada	878	10.8	17.5	162
South Dakota	595	n.a.	17.3	n.a.
South Carolina	2,840	14.3	17.2	120
Nebraska	1,383	9.4	16.9	180
New York	15,286	13.1	16.7	127
Utah	1,546	10.0	16.4	164
Colorado	2,769	13.9	16.3	117
Missouri	4,391	10.7	16.3	152
North Dakota	548	n.a.	15.9	n.a.
Washington	3,808	17.2	15.8	92
Maryland	3,972	8.8	15.5	176
Maine	953	11.0	15.2	138
Ohio	9,356	11.1	15.1	136
Vermont	461	n.a.	15.0	n.a.

States by level of private insurance	Total population (000)	Percentage with public coverage only	Percentage uninsured	Uninsured to public coverage ratio (%)
High level				
Illinois	10,093	13.2	14.7	111
Kansas	2,090	8.9	14.3	161
Virginia	4,799	13.0	13.0	100
Hawaii	833	12.5	12.8	102
Connecticut	2,710	10.7	12.7	119
New Jersey	6,682	10.9	12.3	113
Michigan	8,133	16.1	12.1	75
Massachusetts	5,085	10.1	11.9	118
Pennsylvania	9,925	10.9	11.9	109
Iowa	2,532	11.1	11.6	105
New Hampshire	883	n.a.	11.4	n.a.
Wisconsin	4,143	11.3	10.7	95
Minnesota	3,670	12.9	10.6	82
Rhode Island	824	10.1	8.4	83

SOURCE: Data computed from the Employment Benefit Research Institute tabulations of the March 1987 Current Population Survey, *Source Book of Health Insurance Data*, 1989, pp.13-14.

n.a. = Not ascertained because of the small number of cases in the sample.

The majority of the states with the highest uninsured rates were in the South and West, consistent with the regional distribution described earlier. Mississippi had the highest uninsured rate in the country, with 27 percent of the population under 65, followed closely by Texas and New Mexico. The other extreme of the distribution includes the industrial states and those with a strong union tradition, including Rhode Island (8.4 percent), Minnesota (10.6 percent), Wisconsin (10.7 percent), as well as Iowa, Pennsylvania, Massachusetts, Michigan, and New Jersey (at less than 12 percent).

Coverage by public programs also varies by state. Indiana and Arizona had the lowest rates, at 7.3 and 7.6 percent, respectively. Arizona was the last holdout to join Medicaid, which explains its low participation. The reasons for Indiana's low rate are not apparent. The highest rate of public program participation was 18.3 percent in West Virginia. Michigan was not far behind, at 16.1 percent. In fact, Michigan was the only state among the "high-insurance" group with such a large percentage of public program participation. However, the range of difference in public coverage is narrower than the range of differences in the proportion of persons uninsured.

The ratios of the uninsured to Medicaid beneficiaries among the states were consistent with those observed on a regional level. The states with the highest rates of uninsured had the highest ratios of uninsured to public program beneficiaries. The average ratio of uninsured to public program beneficiaries for the "low-insurance" group was close to 200, about 150 for the mid-level group, and about 100 for the high-level group. This means that in states with low levels of insurance, there were two uninsured for each person on a public program, whereas in states with high levels of insurance, the number of uninsured and those on public programs were evenly matched.

Who Are the Uninsured?

While the data on the profile of those lacking any health care coverage and those on public programs largely reflect the relative sizes of these groups in the population, the other policy-relevant explanation is the observed rate of uninsurance and public program participation for various segments in the population. This information is essential for identifying groups at risk and for assessing the differential risk of lacking health care coverage in the population. Accordingly, analyses of the probability, or risk, of being uninsured for various segments in the population, nationwide and for regions and states, by socio-demographic, employment, and economic characteristics, follow.

Socio-Demographic Differentials

The probability of being uninsured in the United States as a whole is highest among young adults between the ages of 19 and 24. This age group is twice as likely to be uninsured as the general population: nearly one out of three (or 30.2 percent) of those 19 to 24 years of age is uninsured (Table 7). This high uninsured rate is paralleled by a low coverage by public programs, exacerbating the problem faced by this group of young adults.

The next most likely age group to be uninsured is children under 19 years of age. However, public program (primarily Medicaid) participation in this younger age group is rather high, at 12.7 percent. Thus, Medicaid has compensated for some of the deficit in private health insurance coverage among young people in this country. Nevertheless, given that "current benefit levels indicate that, especially for working-age adults and their children, current eligibility for Medicaid is contingent upon virtual destitution" (Johns and Adler 1989), a smaller proportion of Americans with incomes below the poverty line are now covered by Medicaid,[12] and Medicaid spending per child declined from 1978 to 1984 (Johns and Adler 1989, p. 172).

Females have a slightly lower rate of uninsurance than males, in part due to the fact that more of them are covered by Medicaid. While it appears that Medicaid has served as an equalizer for women's insurance protection, spending per AFDC adult also diminished from 1978 to 1984, thereby decreasing the probability that physicians would treat Medicaid beneficiaries.

Being single, divorced, or separated carries a higher probability of being uninsured, as compared with the general population. When looking at these subgroups separately, some important differentials emerge in the relative disadvantage associated with certain groups. For example, approximately one-third of all single individuals are either uninsured or on a public program, with most of them being uninsured. Similarly, a little over 38 percent of divorced or separated persons are in these same categories, again with the largest portion being uninsured. On the other hand, while about a third of the widowed are uninsured or have public coverage, this group has the lowest rate of uninsurance of all adults and the highest rate of public program participation.

Finally, the disadvantage associated with minority status is obvious. Forty-seven percent of blacks and 49 percent of Hispanics are either uninsured or have public coverage only, and they face two-and-one-half times the risk of being uninsured as whites. Blacks are more likely to have public coverage, while Hispanics are more likely to be uninsured.

Overall, families have a 12 percent risk of being uninsured (Table 8). The probability of being uninsured among single-parent families and their dependents is 19.2 percent, about a third higher than families over-all. Single individuals with no dependents face a similar risk. Two-parent families and their dependents are slightly less likely to be uninsured than the population as a whole; households with two or more adults with no dependents are one-third less likely to be uninsured than the general population. All told, the risk of being uninsured increases two times between the household most and least at risk.

The data on socio-demographic characteristics of the uninsured and those on public programs reveal the dynamic relationship between the two conditions. It is clear that were it not for Medicaid, a much larger proportion of the population, including a substantial number of poor women and their dependent children, would be without any health care protection. At the same time, it is obvious that the Medicaid safety net has let a substantial proportion of the poor slip through the holes.

Economic and Employment Differentials

As was the case with the socio-demographic profile, the distribution of the uninsured by these characteristics largely reflects the relative size of each subgroup in the population. For example, while full-time workers have lower rates of uninsurance than part-time workers, they make up a much larger proportion of the uninsured due to the fact there are many more full-time than part-time workers. The earlier distributions described the uninsured, and they are useful in identifying the types of programs that might provide coverage to the largest proportion of the uninsured. Nonetheless, policymakers interested in targeting programs at subpopulations with higher rates of being uninsured require information on the probabilities of uninsurance to provide a clear perspective regarding relative risk.

Those at highest risk of having no health insurance are the unemployed (42 percent) and part-time workers (24.1 percent); workers in small firms employing fewer than 10 individuals (26.3 percent); those who work in personal services (31.5 percent), entertainment (30.6 percent), construction (30.6 percent) or agriculture (29.6 percent); workers who do not belong to a union (16.5 percent); workers who earn less than $5 an hour (30.3 percent) or below $20,000 a year (between 35.4 and 25.8 percent); or those who live at or below the federal poverty line (37.0 percent).

As would be expected in a country that ties health insurance to employment, the full-time employed have the lowest probability of being uninsured, while the unemployed have the highest, over two-and-one-half times that of the overall population (Table 9). Part-time workers are the next most vulnerable, with one-and-one-half times the risk of having no health insurance when compared to the general population, followed closely by the self-employed and those not in the labor force.

In relation to size of firm, the probability of being uninsured increases as the number of employees decreases. In the United States, employees of small firms with less than 10 workers are 75 percent more likely to be uninsured than those in medium firms employing 10 to 100 employees, and almost four-and-one-half times more likely than those in large firms of over 100 employees. The relative disadvantage for employees of small firms is also an absolute disadvantage when comparing the uninsured rates of workers in different-sized firms to the general population. Nationwide, individuals in small firms have one-and-one-half times the likelihood of being uninsured compared to the U.S. population as a whole, while those in large firms are over two-and-one-half times less likely to be uninsured.

Individuals employed in agriculture, construction, personal services, and entertainment all have about twice the risk of being uninsured as the average American, while those in sales and repairs are about 30 percent more likely to be without insurance. Mining, manufacturing, transportation, communication, and utilities, and the professional services industries have about a third lower risk of being uninsured than the average, and public administration and financial services industries have even lower rates of uninsurance.

Workers who are union members are about 70 percent less likely to be uninsured than the general population of working nonmembers, and are two-thirds less likely to be uninsured than the average.

Nationally, families with nonworking adults are only slightly more likely to be uninsured than families with a working adult or the overall population, a fact that reflects Medicare coverage for nonworkers aged 65 or more[13] (Table 8). When considering families whose members are younger than 65, the risk of a family without a working adult is 28.7 percent, almost twice the risk of either families with working adults or the population as a whole.

Generally, one-third of those earning $5 or less an hour are uninsured, twice the rate of both workers who earn $5 to $10 an hour, and the population overall (Table 10). Individuals whose hourly wages exceed $10 an hour are 42 to 66 percent less likely to be uninsured than the national average, and the differential in the probability of being uninsured increases sixfold between the highest and lowest wage earners.

Family income is inversely related to the probability of being uninsured, as is income as a ratio of poverty. Families in the lowest income category, those with annual incomes of $5,000 or less, are six-and-one-half times more likely to be uninsured than those in the highest income bracket of $40,000 or more. Families in the $20,000 to $29,999 category are as likely to be uninsured as the overall population, while those with higher incomes are less likely to have no health insurance than average, and those with lower incomes are more likely to be uninsured. When computed as a ratio to poverty, families with incomes below the poverty line are one-and-one-half times more likely to be uninsured than families with incomes between 100 and 200 percent of poverty, have two-and-one-third times the risk of the overall population, and four times the risk of families with incomes above 200 percent of poverty. Families with incomes between one and two times the poverty level were almost twice as likely to be uninsured as the general population, while those with incomes above 200 percent of poverty were about 40 percent less likely to be uninsured than the general population.

Regional and State Differentials

The risk of being uninsured by region followed a pattern quite similar to the geographic profile presented earlier (Table 11). Those in the West and South had higher probabilities of being uninsured than in the United States as a whole, and individuals living in the Midwest and Northeast had lower probabilities. Altogether, persons living in the West and South were almost 60 percent more likely to be uninsured than those in the East and Midwest.

The reasons for the wide variation between the regions are not clear. Swartz (1989, p. 2) suggested two explanations: limited Medicaid coverage and the lack of a tradition of strong unions in the South and West. While the latter explanation appears plausible, a perusal of the percentages covered by Medicaid does not completely support the hypothesis, since states with the low, mid-, and high levels of private insurance all had similar ranges of public program coverage for their populations (Table 12). If Arizona is removed from the West, the overall regional rates of Medicaid coverage would be comparable (Table 11). An interesting datum is the ratio of the uninsured to Medicaid beneficiaries. The lowest ratios are observed in the Northeast and Midwest, and the highest in the South and West, as follows:

Region	Ratio of Uninsured to Medicaid (expressed as percent)
Northeast	110
Midwest	122
South	166
West	227

Thus, for every 100 persons on Medicaid in the Northeast there were 110 uninsured, whereas in the West this ratio was 227.

Dimensions of the Uninsured Population in Michigan

In Michigan, the Health Insurance Survey of Michigan (HISM) was commissioned by the Governor's Task Force on Access to Health Care to obtain current, accurate, and reliable information on the uninsured, underinsured, and individuals with difficulties obtaining care. Some results from this survey are presented in Tables 13 and 14. For the most part, they are consistent with the national data presented in this chapter. A full report on the findings of HISM was issued by the Task Force (Bashshur, Webb and Homan 1989).

Conclusion

The problem of the uninsured (persons lacking any health care coverage) currently occupies center stage in discussions of health care policy at the federal and state levels. The number of medically uninsured persons has been increasing over the last two decades, and the conscience of the nation dictates that no person should be denied service when facing a legitimate need for care. Despite notable proposals for national health insurance plans to alleviate the problem, pressure has shifted to the states because federal action is not anticipated in the foreseeable future.

The profile of the uninsured reveals that the majority are young, married or single with dependent children, white, work full time and in small firms, and earn less than $10 an hour. The probability of being uninsured is associated with being relatively young, single, divorced or separated, and a member of a minority group. In terms of employment, the probability of being uninsured is associated with being unemployed or being employed part time, in a small firm, and earning low income.

Geographically, the highest rates of uninsurance are found in the South and West and in states with low rates of participation in Medicaid and limited employment in large manufacturing firms with strong traditions of unionization. The great disparity between the regions and the states suggests the need for a federal role in addressing the problem as the equalizer.

Table 13

Probabilities and Percentage Distributions of Individuals With Public Coverage Only or No Insurance, by Selected Socio-Demographic and Economic Characteristics: Michigan, 1989

Population characteristic	Probability of		Percentage distribution[a]	
	Public coverage only (%)	Uninsured (%)	Public coverage only	Uninsured
Total	10.7	10.1	100.0	100.0
Age				
18 and younger	16.1	10.4	46.3	31.9
19-24	8.6	20.9	8.1	21.2
25-64	7.6	9.6	34.4	46.1
65 and older	11.3	0.8	11.2	0.8
Sex				
Male	9.4	10.8	42.4	51.7
Female	12.0	9.4	57.6	48.3
Marital status				
Married	4.5	6.1	18.6	26.8
Single	9.1	22.7	13.7	36.5
Divorced & separated	27.1	11.0	19.0	8.2
Widowed	15.5	5.9	7.0	2.8
Ethnicity				
White	7.0	8.5	53.8	70.3
Black	28.7	15.5	38.2	22.4

SOURCE: Health Insurance Survey of Michigan, 1989.

a. Due to missing data, the percentage distribution figures may not add to 100 percent.

Table 14
Probabilities and Percentage Distribution
of Uninsured Individuals Under 65 Years of Age,
by Economic Variables: Michigan, 1989

Employment characteristic	Probability of being uninsured[a] (%)	Percentage distribution of uninsured[a]
Total	11.2	100.0
Employment status		
Full-time/full-year	8.1	50.6
Part-time/part-year	16.2	21.0
Unemployed	33.8	9.7
Not in labor force	13.6	18.7
Size of firm		
Less than 10 workers	26.5	38.5
10-100 workers	10.6	21.4
Over 100 workers	3.1	11.7
Industry		
Agriculture	28.6	0.8
Mining	33.3	2.9
Construction	22.1	11.9
Manufacturing	2.2	4.4
Transportation & communications	n.a.	n.a.
Sales	16.4	20.0
Financial services	2.6	0.8
Repair services	30.0	2.5
Personal services	48.4	12.5
Professional services	7.5	14.3
Entertainment	6.9	0.4
Public administration	2.2	0.8
Union affiliation		
Member	2.6	5.8
Nonmembers	13.1	65.8

SOURCE: Computed from 1989 HISM data.

NOTE: Working adults are classified according to their own employment characteristics. Non-working spouses classified as not in the labor force. Children, including dependents up to age 25, are classified by the characteristics of the worker. Dependents of couples are classified by the characteristics of the male head of household. Figures do not include individuals with unknown employment status, establishment size, or union membership.

a. Figures may not add to 100 percent because of missing categories.

n.a. = Not ascertained due to small number of cases in the sample.

Since the uninsured are a heterogeneous group, an essential first step for any state addressing the problem of access is the collection of information concerning socio-demographic, economic and employment characteristics of the target population. An example of the nature of such information is provided by the 1989 survey of health insurance coverage in Michigan. Such information can serve as the foundation for rational policy by informing policymakers of the magnitude and distribution of the uninsured in their state, and determining what groups are most at risk.

NOTES

1. For an identification and discussion of the dimensions of access, see Penchansky and Thomas (1981).

2. These figures are from 1987 and 1988 Current Population Survey (CPS) estimates of the number of uninsured. Changes in the number and types of questions on health insurance for the 1988 version resulted in a large disparity between 1987 and 1988 estimates. Estimates of the number of uninsured in 1987 obtained from the National Medical Expenditure Survey (NMES) are almost identical to the 1987 CPS estimates. For more detail, see Swartz (1989); Moyer (1989); and Short, Monheit, and Beauregard (1989).

3. 1977 estimates found in Brown (1988) and Farley (1985). See Note 2 for citations for 1987 estimates.

4. The final data from the March 1988 CPS survey were not made generally available for public use. For information on preliminary data from 1988, see Moyer (1989). Preliminary results of the March 1989 CPS survey can be found in Employee Benefit Research Institute (EBRI 1990).

5. For data on average weekly earnings in current and constant 1977 dollars, see Table 661 in U.S. Bureau of the Census (1989), p. 397.

6. For data on employees average weekly hours, see Table 655 in U.S. Bureau of the Census (1989), p. 404.

7. The U.S. General Accounting Office found that from 1973-1985 there was a 44 percent increase in expenditures, measured in constant dollars; however, all of the expenditure growth occurred during the 1970s. "After Adjusting for Inflation, Essentially No Growth Has Occurred in Medicaid Expenditures During the 1980's." For extended discussion, see Howell, Baugh, and Pine (1988).

8. See the discussion on empirical results, Section A on page 258 in Manning et al. (1987).

9. See "Access to Health Care in the United States: Results of a 1986 Survey" (The Robert Wood Johnson Foundation, Special Report Number Two, 1987), as cited by King (1989).

10. See "Healthy Start Program Evaluation, Preliminary Report" (Massachusetts Department of Public Health, 1988) and "Preventing Low Birthweight: Summary" (Washington, DC: Institute of Medicine, National Academy Press, 1985), p. 50, as cited by King (1989), p. 4.

11. See Table 5 in U.S. General Accounting Office (1990), p. 8.

12. Sixty-three percent of persons with income below the federal poverty line were covered by Medicaid in 1975, as compared with 41 percent in 1986, as reported by King (1989), p. 3.

13. Table 3 in Short, Monheit, and Beauregard (1989), p. 8.

References

Bashshur, R., C. Webb, and R. Homan. 1989. *Health Insurance Survey of Michigan on Access to Health Care.* The Governor's Task Force on Access to Health Care, 2.

Brown, E.R. 1988. "Principles for a National Health Program: Framework for Analysis and Development," *Milbank Quarterly* 66 (4): 573-617.

————. 1989. "Access to Health Insurance in the United States," *Medical Care Review* 46(4): 349-85.

Doyle, P.M. 1985. "Area Wage Surveys Shed Light On Declines In Unionization," *Monthly Labor Review* 108(9): 13-20.

Dunlop, B.D., J.A. Wells, and G.R. Wilensky. 1989. "The Influence of Source of Insurance Coverage on the Health Care Utilization Patterns of the Elderly," *The Journal of Health and Human Resources Administration* 11(3): 285-311.

Employee Benefit Research Institute (EBRI). 1990. "Update: Americans Without Health Insurance," *EBRI Issue Brief* 104 (July).

Farley, P.J. 1985. *Who are the Underinsured?* National Health Care Expenditures Study. Rockville, MD: Public Health Service.

Herz, D.E. 1990. "Worker Displacement in a Period of Rapid Job Expansion: 1983-1987," *Monthly Labor Review* 113(5): 21-33.

Howell, E.M., D.K. Baugh, and P.L. Pine. 1988. "Patterns of Medicaid Utilization and Expenditures in Selected States: 1980-84," *Health Care Financing Review* 10(2): 1-15.

Johns, L. and G.S. Adler. 1989. "Evaluation of Recent Changes in Medicaid," *Health Affairs* 8(2):171-81.

King, M.P. 1989. *Medical Indigence and Uncompensated Health Care Costs.* National Conference of State Legislatures, July.

Kutscher, R.E. and V. Personick. 1986. "Deindustrialization and the Shift to Services," *Monthly Labor Review* 109(6): 2-13.

Manning, W.G., J.P. Newhouse, N. Duan, E.B. Keeler, A. Leibowitz, and M.S. Marquis. 1987. "Health Insurance and the Demand for Medical Care: Evidence from a Randomized Experiment," *The American Economic Review* 77(3): 251-77.

Monheit, A.C. and C.L. Schur. 1988. "The Dynamics of Health Insurance Loss: A Tale of Two Cohorts," *Inquiry* 25 (Summer): 315-27.

Moyer, M.E. 1989. "A Revised Look at the Number of Uninsured Americans," *Health Affairs* (Summer).

Nelson, C. and K. Short. 1990. *Health Insurance Coverage 1986-88,* Bureau of the Census, U. S. Department of Commerce Current Population Reports, Series P-70, No. 17 (March).

Office of National Health Cost Estimates. 1990. "National Health Expenditures, 1988," *Health Care Financing Review* 11(4): 1-41.

Penchansky, R. and W.J. Thomas. 1981. "The Concept of Access: Definition and Relationship to Consumer Satisfaction," *Medical Care* 19 (2): 127-40.

Personick, V. 1987. "Projections 2000: Industry Output and Employment Through the End of the Century," *Monthly Labor Review* 110(9): 25-30.

Renner, C. and V. Navarro. 1989. "Why Is Our Population of Uninsured and Underinsured Persons Growing? The Consequences of the 'Deindustrialization' of America," *Annual Review of Public Health* 10: 85-94.

Ruben, G. 1990. "Collective Bargaining in 1989: Old Problems, New Issues," *Monthly Labor Review* 113(1): 19-29.

Short, P.E. 1988. "Trends in Employee Health Benefits," *Health Affairs* 7: 189.

Short, P.E., A. Monheit, and K. Beauregard. 1989. *A Profile of Uninsured Americans, National Medical Expenditure Survey Research Findings 1.* Rockville, MD: Public Health Service.

Swartz, K. 1989. *The Medically Uninsured: Special Focus on Workers.* Washington, DC: Urban Institute Press.

Swartz, K. and T.D. McBride. 1990. "Spells Without Health Insurance: Distributions of Durations and Their Link to Point-In-Time Estimates of the Uninsured," *Inquiry* 27 (Fall): 281-88.

U.S. Bureau of the Census. 1989. *Statistical Abstract of the United States: 1989,* 109th ed. Washington, DC: Government Printing Office.

U.S. General Accounting Office. 1989. *Health Insurance: An Overview of the Working Uninsured* (HRD-89-45). Washington, DC: U.S. Government Printing Office, February.

_____. 1988. *Health Insurance: A Profile of the Uninsured in Ohio and the Nation* (HRD-88-83). Washington, DC: Government Printing Office, August.

_____. 1990. *A Profile of the Uninsured in Michigan and the United States* (HRD-90-97). Washington, DC: Government Printing Office, May.

World Health Organization. 1978. *Alma Ata 1978: Primary Health Care, No. 1,* Health Care Series, Geneva.

Part II

State Level Policies to Improve Access

3
Universal Health Insurance Coverage Through a Single Public Payer

Andrew J. Hogan
John H. Goddeeris
Michigan State University

Support for a universal health insurance through a single payer grew in the United States during the 1980s (Blendon 1991), especially among public health professionals and labor unions. Recently a number of large corporations have expressed support for the "Canadian Model" of universal health insurance, largely out of their frustration with private efforts to control health care costs (Califano 1989). The two principal motivations for interest in a Canadian-style universal health insurance plan are: (1) to provide access to basic health services as a right of all citizens; and (2) to control health care costs.

This chapter will focus primarily on the first issue of providing access to basic health services for all citizens. The implications of a single-payer public health insurance program for cost containment will be discussed, though not in great detail. It should be noted that the Canadian health insurance system was not designed principally to bring about health care cost containment (Evans 1988), and that the claim that Canada has been significantly more successful than the United States in restraining health expenditure growth has been called into question (Neuschler 1990, pp. 37-46; Goodman and Musgrave 1991, pp. 2-9; for a pro-Canadian view, see Barer, Welch and Antioch 1991). There is no doubt that Canada spends much less on health care than the United States by any measure, or that since the full implementation of universal coverage in the early 1970s health care spending as a share of GNP has grown more slowly there. But this latter result is to some degree due to slower GNP growth in the United States. In *per capita* terms, real personal health expenditures have grown at about the same rate in the two countries during the time that Canada has had universal coverage. Further, Canada enjoys the luxury of using the U.S. health care system as a safety valve when demand exceeds planned capacity.

The U.S. health system is highly decentralized and consumer-driven. For those who can afford health insurance, the system provides very easy access to the latest technology in settings with excellent amenities. While the U.S. health system may not appear rational from a public health perspective, it is highly responsive to the needs of privately insured consumers.

The U.S. health system is clearly undergoing financial distress. Because of the system's decentralized, consumer-driven nature and because poverty, illness, and lack of health insurance tend to cluster in the same population groups, this financial distress is manifested in an increasingly noncompetitive performance in achieving public health objectives compared to other industrialized nations (Bodenheimer 1989, p. 10). Although the causes are undoubtedly complex and go beyond the reach of medical care alone, much of the poor public health performance can be attributed to the lack of ready access by one-quarter to one-third of the population to routine preventive health services and primary medical care. This lack of access is due largely to a lack of personal financial resources, expressed most often as a lack of adequate health insurance coverage (Pepper Commission 1990, pp. 33-35). Included in this subpopulation are those covered by Medicaid, which in most states pays providers such low rates that recipients frequently encounter difficulty in finding providers who will accept them, particularly in specialties like obstetrics (Pepper Commission 1990, pp. 30-31). Growth in the number of uninsured results from reduced health insurance coverage rates by both private employers and by Medicaid (Piacentini and Cerino 1990, pp. 246, 352).

Reductions in insurance coverage for the working poor may be a reflection of the fact that their real incomes have not increased while health care costs have soared (Piacentini and Cerino 1990; Peterson 1991). The working poor may have accepted a lack of health insurance in preference to further wage cuts. And as both the willingness and ability of many working class households to increase tax contributions waned during the 1980s, funding of public health insurance programs (Medicaid, Medicare, Veterans Administration) has not kept pace with increases in health care costs or with the growth of the poverty and near-poverty populations. The combination of large numbers of uninsured and underfunded public programs has shifted much of the burden for the sizable real growth in personal health expenditures onto private insurers and self-insured employers and union trusts. Consequently, employers and workers have experienced disproportionately large increases in health care costs (Levit and Cowan 1990). This has, in turn, engendered risk-avoidance maneuvering in the private insurance market, especially the market for individual and small business policies. These markets constantly churn as insurers and insureds attempt to shift risk onto each other, illustrating some of the classic symptoms of insurance market failure described by Rothschild and Stiglitz (1976).

Thus, while we may be skeptical that a single-payer universal health insurance plan could by itself retard the growth of health care costs due to population aging, technological change, or the deeply held predilection of the American public for medical miracles, such a plan could reduce the administrative and transaction costs associated with the current health insurance market and could provide a mechanism through which public health goals could be given some ascendancy over individual medical consumerism. It goes without saying that a universal health insurance plan would alleviate problems of access to basic health care that arise from the lack of financial resources at the household level.

This chapter briefly discusses the implications for health care costs of a state-initiated program of universal coverage. There are many open questions here, but it is not realistic to expect such a program to substantially slow the growth of costs in the near future. The heart of the analysis considers the likely redistributional effects of a move to universal coverage, including illustrative quantitative estimates for Michigan. A Canadian-style system is likely to redistribute income toward the currently uninsured poor and away from those in the upper tail of the income distribution. When initiated by a single state, it would also risk losing significant subsidies built into the federal tax system. Even a state plan providing only basic coverage and financed in a way that retains federal subsidies would have important redistributional effects.

Universal Health Coverage and Health Care Costs

Comparisons with Canada and other countries around the world have raised hopes in the United States that a state system of universal coverage could improve public health outcomes while actually reducing the total cost of health care. There are three main arguments for this view: (1) a single-payer system would substantially reduce administrative costs; (2) a single payer could exert greater control over fees for services and impose a more rational pattern of investment in capital and equipment on the industry; and (3) universal coverage would lead to a more efficient utilization of services by the currently uninsured that would reduce the total cost of their health care. With regard to the last point, it is tempting to think that better coverage for the uninsured would lead to healthier lifestyles, greater use of preventive care, and earlier treatment when acute problems arise, and that all of these things would translate into lower, not higher, total health care costs. The available evidence indicates, however, that the uninsured use less care than those who are insured and have similar characteristics (Long and Rodgers 1990). The natural inference is that improving their access to care will, on net, increase their consumption.

While each of these arguments for the cost-saving potential of universal coverage is important and merits continued research, it is unlikely that a move to such a system in the United States would reduce the growth of health care spending in the near term, particularly if enacted by a single state rather than the national government. Let us consider arguments (1) and (2) in somewhat more detail, focusing particularly on how they apply to a state-initiated system.

Administrative Costs

One appealing argument for a system of universal coverage is the potential for enormous savings in administrative costs. It has been suggested that more than half of the difference in *per capita* costs between the American and Canadian health care systems may be accounted for by higher administrative cost in the United States (Evans et al. 1989; Himmelstein and Woolhandler 1986). A single public payer has no need to incur many of the costs that competing private insurance plans must bear. These include all of the costs of marketing, of screening potential enrollees in order to set appropriate premiums, of determining appropriate differentials in premiums for different risk classes of enrollees, of determining eligibility when claims are paid, of coordination of benefits when members of the same household are covered by more than one plan, as well as the additional costs arising when individuals change their coverage. Even the collection of premiums is likely to be much less costly when carried out as part of a state tax system already in place than when spread across many competing insurance firms.

More important are the additional costs related to administration of the health care system incurred by health care providers and consumers. Doctors and hospitals bear a heavy burden of administrative cost in dealing with large numbers of different insurers, in determining the eligibility of patients, and in direct billing and collections. Consumers and their employers incur costs associated with comparison of plans in making decisions about which to choose. The considerable resources devoted in the current system to the zero-sum game of cost-shifting would presumably be saved in a universal system.

It is important to understand, however, that Canada's system has a number of features that contribute to its very low level of administrative cost, and that elimination of any of these features would correspondingly reduce administrative cost savings. The Canadian system provides the same coverage to everyone in a province through a single payer, with minimal cost-sharing by patients, no balance-billing by providers, and no supplemental private insurance coverage for services covered under the public system.

With the federally funded Medicare program already in place and providing health coverage to the elderly and disabled in the United States, it is unlikely that a state would want to displace that coverage and lose federal funds. Thus, at least Medicare (and other federal health care programs through the Department of Defense and Veterans Administration) would remain in place, as would private insurance coverage supplemental to Medicare, unless it is included as part of the state program. If individuals are to be allowed a choice among competing plans, or if the universal plan provides only basic coverage that may be supplemented privately, or if consumer cost-sharing is relied upon (as a way to limit use of services or to reduce the central plan's share of cost), administrative cost savings would fall considerably.

Administrative costs are also lower in Canada because less attempt is made in that system to track the costs of individual patients or to monitor the appropriateness of care (Neuschler 1990). Unless these efforts are abandoned in the United States (which seems unlikely even if a system of universal coverage is adopted), they will remain a source of greater administrative overhead. Finally, it should be understood that to realize administrative savings would require the elimination of existing jobs in the health insurance industry and elsewhere in the health care system. Canada and other countries have never had the enormous commitment of resources to health insurance administration that the United States has, and thus did not face the problem of scaling it back.

Fees, Budgets, and a Single Payer

Undoubtedly, some of Canada's success in keeping health care costs below those in the U.S. derives from the ability of a single payer to control physicians' fees and hospital budgets. These are determined by a process of negotiation involving medical societies, provincial hospital associations, and departments of health (and ultimately the provincial legislatures). In contrast to the very decentralized and open-ended U.S. system, this process does place limits on total health spending, but it does so in a rather unsophisticated way. There is no guarantee that the total level of spending is in any sense socially optimal, or even that the limited resources going to health care are used in the most efficient way possible.

How well the Canadian system of budgeting would work in the United States, and particularly for a single state on its own, is an open question. As Victor Fuchs (1986) has emphasized, total health care expenditures may be viewed as the product of costs per service and volume of services, and both elements must be controlled to contain expenditure growth over the long run. With regard to physicians' services, Canada has had less success limiting volume of services than controlling fees. Total hospital budgets are set, but as a result some health services are apparently not as readily available to middle-income and upper-income

Canadians as to their U.S. counterparts (Goodman and Musgrave 1991, pp. 17-18; Rublee 1991).

It is often said that U.S. consumers will not tolerate the waiting or denial of services which the Canadians are said to have learned to accept. If that is so, the potential for constraining the use of medical services through a single payer may be limited. A single state would also have much less monopoly power in dealing with physicians than would the U.S. government or even a Canadian province. Physicians' fees (or, more important, physicians' total incomes) could not be kept far below those in other states without prompting extensive out-migration of doctors and consequent access problems due to physician shortages.

Political Concerns

Whether resources devoted to health care would increase or decrease in the aggregate with the establishment of state-financed universal coverage depends to a great extent on the political willingness to constrain costs. Under any reasonable cost-containment scenario, it seems certain that the distribution of resources would be greatly affected. The current U.S. health care system is oriented to satisfying the demands of the privately insured employee or retiree, with the needs of public-pay-only patients being met for the most part as either volume filler or as part of a social mission. Under a single-payer system, all patients provide an equal opportunity for financial gain or loss. Barring large copayments which the poor would be unable to pay, some resources now devoted to serving the privately insured would shift toward population groups that are currently underserved. This would be especially true if the universal health insurance plan prohibits private rivals or supplements, as is the case in Canada. If the benefit plan is reasonably comprehensive with minimal copayments and if private health insurance for services covered in the national health plan is prohibited, then a significant redistribution of resources would likely take place. If the national health plan resembles the U.S. Medicare program, where Medicare-only coverage is tantamount to being underinsured and where most middle-income and upper-income retirees have supplemental private insurance, then the redistribution would be considerably moderated.

If cost containment were a sustainable political goal in a universal health plan, then we could expect those who are now well-insured to see a reduction in their real coverage (access to services on demand) over time. Depending on the financing mechanism used, that same group of upper-middle and upper-income voters is likely to be asked to bear a larger share of the cost than it currently does. The political feasibility of simultaneously reducing coverage and increasing the cost burden for a large block of relatively affluent voters seems dubious and casts doubt on the potential of a state-initiated universal health care system to truly contain costs.

Given the fate of the Medicare Catastrophic Coverage legislation with its redistributional premium structure, the political feasibility of a single-payer universal health plan which also truly constrains the normal growth in personal health expenditures is doubtful.[1]

Distributional Effects of Universal Coverage
An Illustration Using Michigan Data

Any universal health care plan implemented by a state may create major changes in the distribution of health care use and in how the costs are borne. In this section we analyze the distributional effects of two illustrative approaches to universal health care, using data from Michigan. Our analysis requires us to make a number of assumptions, which could be tested more carefully against empirical data. More study is clearly desirable before implementation of any plan. At least some of the patterns we identify are strong enough, however, that we doubt that they would be substantially altered in a more comprehensive study.

The two approaches to universal coverage we consider are: (1) a Canadian-style system, with a single public payer supported by income taxes, excluding all forms of private coverage, and with minimal copayments; and (2) a mixed public-private option in which there is limited universal coverage similar to that provided in the current U.S. Medicare program, with possible private supplementary insurance. Both approaches exclude populations currently receiving health care coverage through federal programs (Medicare, the Departments of Defense and Veterans Affairs). Our rationale is that a state would not want to forgo federal funding and would therefore expect such individuals to retain their current coverage.

Our main focus is on the distributional implications of alternative financing mechanisms, and we downplay other possible effects of a system of universal coverage. We do assume some increase in utilization of care for the currently uninsured, but no effects for others. Costs per unit of care are treated as the same under all options, and no administrative savings are incorporated. Proponents of universal coverage may perceive this as biased against their view, but we consider the cost-containment potential of a universal system to be sufficiently uncertain that our assumptions are a reasonable baseline.

The Current System

To provide a background for the analysis, we begin by describing the distributional impacts of the current system in Michigan. Data on population, income, and insurance coverage are taken from the 1988 Current Population Survey and its supplement on health insurance. These data refer to conditions in 1987. We divide the population into family "insurance units"[2] and array the families by income as a percent of the federal poverty standard. Income is gross money income before taxes and including transfer payments. It does not include the value of fringe benefits, such as employer-provided health insurance. For the value of health care utilized we use 1987 national *per capita* personal health care expenditures (Piacentini and Cerino 1990, p. 160) of $1,726. This *per capita* expenditure is adjusted by a factor of 1.2142 for adults or 0.7041 for children, reflecting relative *per capita* expenditures in the Michigan Medicaid Program for its Aid to Families with Dependent Children population. We adjusted health expenditures by uninsured households to 42 percent of the level of insured households based on data from the Survey of Income and Program Participation (Long and Rodgers 1990; CBO 1991). We also identify as "underinsured" those whose family income was less than 200 percent of the poverty standard and who purchased nongroup health insurance or a group plan for which no employer made a contribution. Our expectation is that insurance coverage is usually quite limited in these cases. We treat consumption of the underinsured as midway between the uninsured and the insured. Lacking sufficient data to do otherwise, we make the simplifying assumptions that medical care use among the other insured does not vary with the type (public vs. private) or comprehensiveness of coverage. In reality, private coverage tends to be less extensive for those at lower incomes and this probably restrains their utilization relative to those with more complete coverage.

In Figure 1 we summarize how the use of health care and the burden of paying for it are currently spread across income classes in Michigan. The bottom (negative) half of the figure depicts health care use. The height of the bar for each income group reflects the amount of health care utilized by the income group, which is determined by the size of the population in the group, the percent who are children, and the percent who are uninsured. We have distinguished public and private utilization. Public utilization is care paid by the Medicaid program. Not surprisingly, it is concentrated at the low end of the income distribution. It may be more surprising that even in the group below the poverty line, less than half of care used is provided by Medicaid.

The top (positive) half of Figure 1 shows how much health care is paid for in each income group. A group may not pay for all the care it uses because some is publicly financed, and some is "uncompensated." We mean by uncompensated any excess in the cost of providing care over the direct payments made by the recipient or any third party. In our analysis uncompensated care is generated by Medicaid, which is assumed to reimburse for only 75 percent of the cost of care for its beneficiaries, and by the uninsured and underinsured. Of course, it is possible that some groups pay for more care than they use, if they pay taxes to support Medicaid or if costs of uncompensated care are shifted to them. Some costs of care are also shifted to out-of-state taxpayers through federal tax subsidies.

In allocating the cost of care, we attribute to each family:

> *Out-of-Pocket Costs:* Out-of-pocket costs were calculated for all as 18 percent of the value of total health care utilized, based on data from the national health accounts (Levit and Cowan 1990). It is likely that this percentage varies with insurance coverage and

Figure 1
1987 Michigan Health Use and Payments
by Income Class and Payment Source

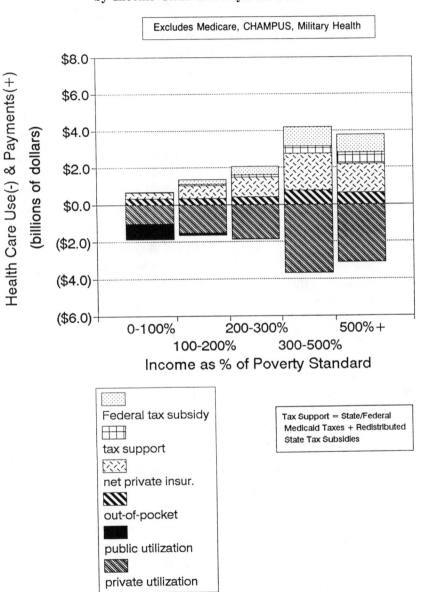

Excludes Medicare, CHAMPUS, Military Health

Legend:
- Federal tax subsidy
- tax support
- net private insur.
- out-of-pocket
- public utilization
- private utilization

Tax Support = State/Federal Medicaid Taxes + Redistributed State Tax Subsidies

income, so that this is an area where better data could improve the precision of the estimates. The remaining care used by the uninsured is uncompensated. For the underinsured, we assume that half of care is covered by insurance, and the remainder after out-of-pocket payments is uncompensated. The broad income groupings that we use also mask the fact that out-of-pocket payments are highly variable within these groups (particularly for the uninsured), depending on the need for care.

Net Private Insurance: This is the cost of its private health insurance, excluding any amount of subsidy through the tax system. Even if insurance is employer-provided, we treat it as though it substitutes for higher wages, so that its cost is borne by the employee. This assumption is standard in the health economics literature, and is discussed in chapter 8 of this volume. For an insured family, the gross cost of health insurance is taken to be the value of health care used but not paid for out-of-pocket (half the value of health care used for the underinsured), plus an imputation for the cost of uncompensated care. In effect we assume that if there were no uncompensated care, insurance premiums in the aggregate would be lower by the current cost of that care.

To deal with the tax subsidy, we compute the taxes an employee *would have paid* on the gross value of employer-provided health insurance if it were treated as taxable income. This includes all FICA[3] taxes, and state and federal income taxes. Tax subsidies for health insurance and health services are calculated based on the family's 1987 marginal tax rate: 14.3 percent FICA (for earnings under $43,000), 0 – 38.5 percent federal income tax,[4] 4.6 percent state income tax. The marginal rate appropriate to the family's taxable income and earnings was multiplied by the value of the family's private health insurance coverage to produce a tax subsidy.[5] The net cost of health insurance is the value of the premium minus the reduction in taxes that results from taking compensation in this form rather than as taxable wages.

Tax Support: Medicaid is tax-supported, with state and federal dollars. The costs of tax subsidies for health insurance are also borne by taxpayers. State Medicaid dollars and state tax subsidies must be paid by Michigan taxpayers, so these costs must be distributed back to Michigan households. State contributions to the Medicaid program and the costs of financing state income tax subsidies for employer-sponsored health insurance were allocated equally to the state sales tax (assumed to be proportioned to total family income) and the state income tax, based on state taxable family income. Federal contributions to the Medicaid program were raised from federal taxable family income at the average marginal rate of 20 percent. The costs of federal spending and tax subsidies, however, are borne by taxpayers throughout the United States. We attribute the federal share of Medicaid to Michigan taxpayers, but treat the federal tax subsidies as shifted to out-of-state taxpayers.[6]

Out-of-pocket costs, net private insurance, and tax support correspond to the first three segments of the top bars in Figure 1. The last segment allocates by income class the federal tax subsidy for employer-provided health insurance. We regard the burden of the subsidy as being borne by out-of-state taxpayers.

Figure 1 shows that the value of health care utilized exceeds the amount paid for at all levels of income. Federal tax subsidies make this possible. The subsidies are unimportant for low-income households, but the poor receive more care than they pay for because of Medicaid coverage and uncompensated care. Higher-income taxpayers must support this care for the poor, but what they pay is not as large as the federal subsidies they receive for their own care. The current system is progressive in the sense that the ratio of payments to health care use rises somewhat with income.

Figure 2 breaks apart the components of tax support in Figure 1 and allows us to look more closely at Michigan's subsidies to health care and financing of Medicaid. Subsidies through the state income tax system must be borne by state taxpayers. Figure 2 shows that these have relatively little redistributive effect across income classes, because those who receive the subsidies to a large degree also pay to refinance them.

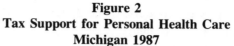

Figure 2
Tax Support for Personal Health Care
Michigan 1987

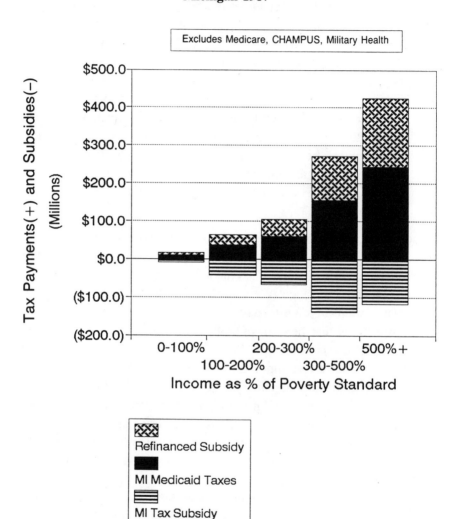

Among families at the same income, the subsidies do favor those with employer-provided health insurance over others. Not surprisingly, tax support for Medicaid comes heavily from households with relatively high incomes.

The Canadian Model

In analyzing a Canadian-style state health plan, we assume that the state is able to retain current federal Medicaid dollars, but that the remaining health care utilization is financed entirely through a nearly threefold increase in the state's flat rate income tax. Health care utilization (displayed in the bottom half of Figure 3) changes from the current system only for those currently uninsured or underinsured. Health care use increases for the uninsured to the level of the rest of the population, more than doubling their medical care consumption. Even this increase in use may understate the benefit of the state plan to the uninsured, as the state plan ends their dependence on uncompensated care, the availability of which is always uncertain and for which quality may be low. In modeling the current system, the underinsured had been treated as consuming medical care at a level half way between the uninsured and the insured. Health care use by the underinsured is therefore also assumed to increase somewhat under the state health plan. In all, these changes represent a 15 percent increase in total health care utilization.

The top bars in Figure 3 show the distribution of the costs of care under this plan. The Canadian-style plan eliminates health insurance as an employee benefit, and we assume that for those with employer-provided coverage wages rise by the employer cost of that coverage (this is implied by the assumption that the cost of health insurance is borne by the worker). However, families now bear a cost through the taxes they pay to finance the state health plan. The bars are divided into three segments. The first is labeled "Current Taxes" and reflects taxes that support the current Medicaid program. We allocate these to income classes exactly as we did for the current system. The second segment shows new state income taxes needed, allocated to taxpayers in each income class.

Figure 3
Health Expenditures and Income Taxes
Canadian-Style Public Health Insurance

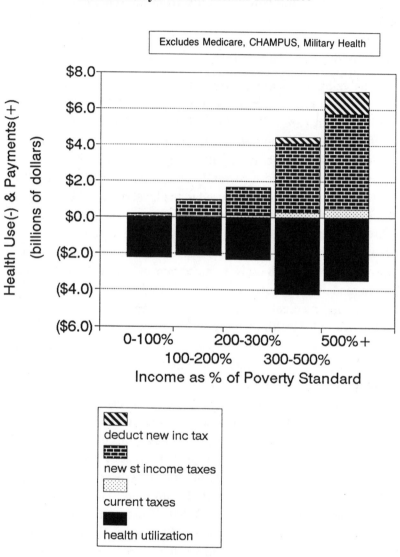

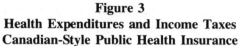

From a state's perspective, a major drawback to an income tax-financed universal health plan is the increase in federal tax liabilities for state residents, as the federal subsidies to employer-provided coverage are forgone. Not all federal subsidies would be lost, however. For those who itemize deductions on their federal returns, higher state taxes are deductible from federal taxable income. In effect, the federal treasury bears a share of each itemizing family's state income tax, equal to the federal marginal tax rate.

The third segment in the top of Figure 3 indicates in each group the portion of higher state taxes shifted to out-of-state taxpayers via deductibility. We calculate this by taking into account federal marginal tax rates and the share of taxpayers in each group who are itemizers (using national averages on itemizing by income in 1987, from U.S. Department of Treasury 1989, Table 1). This segment is small enough to be imperceptible in the figure up to 300 percent of poverty (in the 200-300 percent group it reaches only $48 million).[7] It grows much larger in the highest-income groups, even in relation to new state taxes, for two reasons: higher-income taxpayers face higher marginal tax rates, and they are much more likely to be itemizers.

Compared with the current system, the distribution of the cost is borne more heavily by the higher-income groups under the Canadian-style plan. The Michigan income tax is a flat rate tax, with a personal exemption of $1,600 per member of the household. The exemptions make taxes paid a smaller share of income for those of the low end of the distribution. Because of low tax contributions and the elimination of out-of-pocket payments for their own care, those at the low end of the distribution bear a much smaller portion of the cost than they do currently. For those with incomes up to 200 percent of the poverty level, the ratio of contributions to health care use is significantly lower under the Canadian model than under the current system. The two systems are approximately the same between 200 and 300 percent of poverty, and the ratio becomes much larger for the Canadian model at higher incomes. The higher overall ratio for the Canadian model reflects the loss of federal subsidies, a point to which we will return.

Of course, a state system providing this type of coverage does not have to be financed in this way, and other financing mechanisms (for example, income-based premiums) could have different distributional consequences. Any system that effectively exempts those at low incomes from bearing the costs of their care will, however, involve significant redistributions.

Limited Public Coverage With Private Supplementation

Our alternative version of universal coverage is rather different from the Canadian-style plan. We assume that all are guaranteed limited coverage along the lines of the federal Medicare program (coverage for hospital and physician care, with some limits and cost-sharing), which may then be supplemented with private coverage. Roughly in keeping with Medicare, we assume that the public insurance covers half of the cost of care for a typical household. This coverage is financed through a flat-rate payroll tax on the earnings of all workers, with a ceiling on the amount of payroll tax owed by any individual. The particular form of the payroll tax used in our analysis is an 8.5 percent tax on the first $30,000 of earnings. This combination is sufficient to raise the needed revenue. A higher ceiling would make it possible to reduce the rate somewhat.

To analyze the distribution of health care use and costs under this approach, we must make some additional assumptions concerning whether or not basic public coverage is supplemented with private insurance. We assume that persons currently eligible for Medicaid would be covered fully (basic plus supplemental coverage) through the state/federal Medicaid program. Anyone currently covered by private insurance is assumed to retain it to supplement the public program and cover the other half of medical costs. The supplemental private coverage is assumed to be of the same type as is currently held: group or individual, employer-provided or individually purchased. Those who are currently uninsured do not supplement, and therefore are responsible for half of their health care expenses out-of-pocket. Those in this group with incomes below 200 percent of poverty pay out-of-pocket for 18 percent of what insurance does not cover (as we assume they do in the current system) and default on the remainder. Some uncompensated care thus remains in the system. Its cost is borne in the premiums of supplemental private insurance. As for the payroll tax, it is assumed to be borne by workers. For those who had not been receiving a health benefit in 1987, this means that their earnings fall to offset the amount of payroll tax paid by the employer. Most of the earnings are lost to workers in households with incomes below 200 percent of the poverty standard, roughly 7 percent of the current earnings of workers without employer-provided health insurance.

Figure 4 presents the distribution of health care expenditures and supporting state payroll taxes (8.5 percent) under a mixed public-private state health insurance plan. Redistribution under the mixed plan is not as marked as in the single-payer income tax-supported approach. However, a significant amount of redistribution of health resources would take place, and in a form similar to that of mandated benefits for all employers (see chapter 4 in this volume). Payroll tax financing, as proposed for our second approach, has one distinct advantage over the use of an income tax. The payroll tax would be treated as a business expense and not part of an employee's taxable income. The practical advantage of the payroll tax approach becomes evident when it is recognized that, without federal cooperation, the increase in federal taxes due to the rise in taxable income occasioned by the loss of employee health benefits under a Canadian-style health plan could be 10 percent of total personal health care costs.

Figure 5 summarizes the distributional effects of the current system as compared with the two versions of universal coverage we are considering. For each system and each income class it shows the ratio of net contributions—all payments for health care, netting out subsidies and including taxes—to use of health care. Figure 5 clearly shows that both versions of universal coverage would redistribute resources from the top of the income distribution (primarily those at more than 500 percent of poverty) to those at or near the bottom. In both universal systems those in poverty pay very little for the care they receive, while high-income families pay for more than the cost of their care. The Canadian model, with the open-ended income tax financing we have assumed, is the most redistributive.

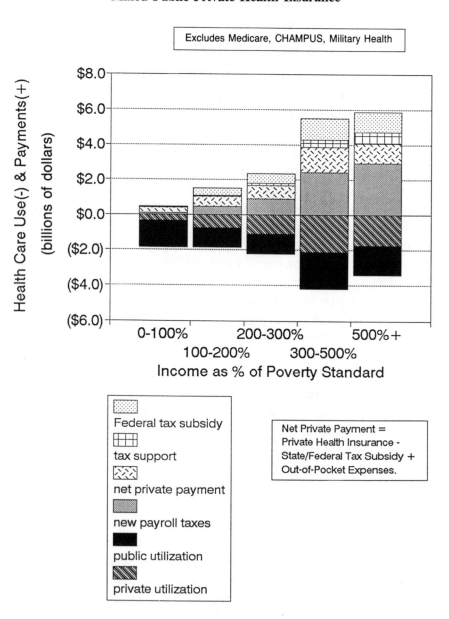

Figure 4
Michigan Health Expenditures and Payroll Taxes
Mixed Public-Private Health Insurance

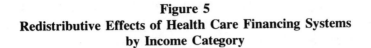

Figure 5
Redistributive Effects of Health Care Financing Systems
by Income Category

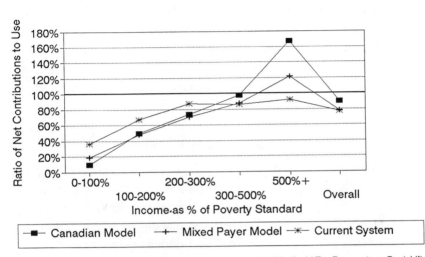

Net Contribution = Private Health Insurance + State/Federal Medicaid Tax Payments + Costshift +
Out-of-Pocket - State/Federal Employee Health Insurance Tax Subsidies +
Redistributed State Health Insurance Tax Subsidies

At the right end of Figure 5 is the overall or average ratio of net contributions to use for each system. It is less than 100 percent in each case because of federal tax subsidies. The overall ratio is the same for the mixed-payer model and the current system at about 75 percent, but the Canadian model sacrifices substantial federal subsidies and the ratio rises to 85 percent. Not shown in Figure 5 is an overall increase in health care expenditures from about $12.4 billion under the current system to $13.8 billion under the mixed model to $14.3 billion under the Canadian system, due to the increased access to care by the uninsured and underinsured.

Concluding Remarks

Clearly, if a state must go-it-alone in a noncooperative federal environment, the mixed-payer system discussed here, along with the mandated-benefit approach discussed in chapter 4, has significant cost advantages. While the mixed-payer and mandated-benefit approaches have been identified as having weak cost-containment potential (Aaron 1991), even the most optimistic proponents of the Canadian-style single-payer health plan will probably be hard pressed to argue that their plans can expand access and reduce costs while overcoming a 10 percent federal income and payroll tax surcharge. Without some cooperation from the federal government on recovery of additional federal income and FICA payroll tax revenues, state-sponsored, income tax-supported health plans appear to be too costly.

Even the modest level of redistribution of health resources involved in the mixed-payer model could make this approach infeasible in the current political climate (Blendon 1991). For those with incomes greater than five times the poverty level, the mixed-payer scenario looks precariously like the Medicare Catastrophic Coverage debacle, where wealthy Medicare beneficiaries were asked to pay actuarially unfair premiums to pay for increased coverage for low-income beneficiaries. Even though the catastrophic coverage still left the wealthy beneficiaries with an overall net subsidy for their full Medicare coverage, they rebelled and successfully forced Congress to repeal the legislation. This lesson will not be lost on state legislators considering either the mixed-payer or the single-payer model.

Examination of the consequences of the single public payer health plan enacted by an individual state brings into sharp contrast the contradictory health care tax and expenditure policies adopted and maintained by state and federal governments in the United States. At a time when state and federal governments have searched ever more aggressively for effective cost-containment strategies and have faced dire fiscal restraints leading to substantial underfunding of major public health insurance programs (and increasingly destabilizing cost-shifting onto private payers), these same units of government are providing ever more subsidies to middle-income and upper-income health insurance policyholders, effectively blunting the demand-side discipline of the market.

Ironically, inaction at the federal level maintains in place a federal tax code which is a formidable obstacle for any state wishing, through a Canadian-style public health insurance model, to bring its population face-to-face with the complete cost of health care, to be paid with highly distasteful income taxes. In the policy experiments reported here, a state government wishing to go-it-alone would almost certainly choose against creating an income and payroll tax windfall for an uncooperative federal government and would probably choose the mixed public-private payer model (or the mandated-benefits approach discussed in chapter 4). However, the mixed-payer model has the effect of increasing total health care tax subsidies,[8] diluting any discipline the demand side of the market might bring to bear on the gap between the growth of *per capita* income and the growth of *per capita* health expenditures. It appears then that fundamental reforms may require the federal government to reassess the *ad hoc* and perhaps outdated policy implemented after World War II of treating employer-provided health insurance as a business expense and not part of taxable compensation.

NOTES

1. Blendon (1991) provides background on American preferences for redistributive health care financing policies and the failure of Medicare catastrophic coverage legislation.

2. Households can contain individuals who cannot be covered under a typical family health insurance policy, i.e., adult children of the head of household or spouse. Households with these kinds of members were broken into insurance units, i.e., familial groups which could be covered by standard health insurance policies.

3. FICA payroll contributions are not considered by all as a tax because, in principle, social security benefits are linked to individual contributions. However, the pay-as-you-go financing used for both social security payments and Medicare means that most current contributions are spent in the same year they are collected and almost always before the individual contributor could make a claim on them. Payment of current FICA payroll taxes may create a moral obligation on a future generation of workers to provide an adequate level of contributions toward the retirement of the current cohort of workers. Nonetheless, we consider the marginal FICA contributions which workers would make on the value of their health benefits, were they to become taxable, to be unrelated for all practical purposes to future social security income, i.e., we consider them to be a tax.

4. Here we calculate the federal marginal income tax rate that would apply if the household did not itemize deductions. This overstates the marginal rate for some itemizers, but we expect this to be a relatively minor source of error. This analysis takes no account of the medical deduction on the federal income tax. That deduction can reduce the price of medical care by a percentage equal to a family's federal marginal tax rate, but only for those who itemize deductions, and only for that portion of medical expenses in excess of 7.5 percent of income. The income restriction severely limits the use of the deduction. Nationally in 1987, only 5 percent of returns claimed the deduction at all, and the total amount deducted was only .6 percent of all income reported (U.S. Department of Treasury, 1989).

5. This treatment of tax subsidies ignores the fact that medical care is excluded from the base of the state's sales tax. This sales tax exclusion encourages consumption of medical care relative to other goods, although it is by no means the only major exclusion from the sales tax base in Michigan or most other states. See chapter 7 in this volume for further discussion.

6. Of course, Michigan taxpayers bear, in an analogous way, some of the costs of health care in all other states. But these costs cannot be controlled by state policies, and therefore are unchanged under any of the options we consider. As we will show, a move to a state health care system could forfeit federal subsidies to Michigan, but Michigan taxpayers would continue to subsidize health care in other states.

7. The increase in the state income tax would surely induce some nonitemizers to switch to itemizing, so our analysis understates to some degree the share of cost shifted out-of-state.

8. While the net contribution to use ratio is the same under the mixed payer model, total use rises, 25 percent of which is financed by state and federal tax subsidies.

References

Aaron, H.J. 1991. "The Worst Health Care Reform Plan . . . . Except for All the Others," *Challenge* 34(6): 61-63.

Barer, M., W.P. Welch and L. Antioch. 1991. "Canadian/U.S. Health Care: Reflections on the HIAA's Analysis," *Health Affairs* 10: 229-36.

Blendon, R.J. 1991. "Health Services Research: Implications for Policy, Management and Clinical Practice." Presidential Address to the Eighth Annual Meeting of the Association for Health Services Research, San Diego, CA, June.

Bodenheimer, T.S. 1989. "Payment Mechanisms and a National Health Program," *Medical Care Review* 46(1): 3-43.

Califano, J.A. 1989. "Billions Blown on Health," *New York Times,* April 11.

CBO (Congressional Budget Office). 1991. *Selected Options for Expanding Health Insurance Coverage.* Washington, DC: U.S. Congress.

Evans, R. 1988. Presentation at Summer Meeting of the Board of Trustees of Blue Cross and Blue Shield of Michigan, Harbor Springs, MI, July.

Evans, R. et al. 1989. "Controlling Health Expenditures: The Canadian Reality," *New England Journal of Medicine* 320: 571-77.

Fuchs, V.R. 1986. "Has Cost Containment Gone Too Far?" *The Milbank Quarterly* 64(3): 186-196.

GAO (U.S. General Accounting Office). 1991. *Canadian Health Insurance: Lesson for the United States.* GAO/HRD-91-90, June.

Goodman, J.C. and G.L. Musgrave. 1991. *Twenty Myths About National Health Insurance.* Dallas, TX: National Center for Policy Analysis, Policy Report No. 128.

Himmelstein, D.V. and S. Woolhandler. 1986. "Cost Without Benefit: Administrative Waste in U.S. Health Care," *New England Journal of Medicine* 314: 441-45.

Leibowitz, A., W.G. Manning, E.B. Keeler, et al. 1985. "The Effect of Cost Sharing on the Use of Medical Services by Children." Santa Monica, CA: Rand Corporation Report R-3287-HHS.

Levit, K.R. and C.A. Cowan. 1990. "The Burden of Health Care Costs: Business, Household, and Governments." *Health Care Financing Review* 12(2): 127-137.

Long, S.H. and J. Rodgers. 1990. "The Effects of Being Uninsured on Health Care Service Use Estimates from the Survey of Income and Program Participation." Survey of Income and Program Participation (SIPP) Working Paper No. 9012, Bureau of the Census.

Neuschler, E. 1990. *Canadian Health Care: The Implications of Public Health Insurance.* Washington, DC: Research Bulletin of the Health Insurance Association of America.

Pepper Commission (U.S. Bipartisan Commission on Comprehensive Health Care). 1990. *Final Report: A Call for Action.* Washington, DC: U.S. Government Printing Office.

Peterson, W.C. 1991. "The Silent Depression," *Challenge* 34(4): 29-34.

Piacentini, J.S. and T.J. Cerino. 1990. *EBRI Data Book on Employee Benefits.* Washington, DC: Employee Benefit Research Institute.

Rothschild, M. and J. Stiglitz. 1976. "Equilibrium in Competitive Insurance Markets: An Essay on the Economics of Imperfect Information," *Quarterly Journal of Economics* 4: 629-650.

Rublee, D.A. 1991. "Can We Develop an Equitable System in an Era of Limited Health Care Resources." In *The Future of Health Care: Public Concerns and Policy Trends.* Boston: Health Data Corporation.

Scheiber, G.J. 1990. "Health Expenditures in Major Industrialized Countries, 1960-87, *Health Care Financing Review* 11(4): 159-167.

U.S. Department of Treasury, Internal Revenue Service. 1989. *Statistics of Income Bulletin,* Publication 1136.

4

Combining Private Insurance with Public Programs to Achieve Universal Coverage

John H. Goddeeris
Michigan State University

For many who embrace universal health insurance as an objective, a tax-financed state plan that would cover all residents is simply too radical a restructuring of the current health care system. In 1987, the share of personal health expenditures accounted for by private health insurance amounted to about 3.1 percent of gross national product, or $552 per capita (Letsch, Levit, and Waldo 1988). This is more than half of the amount raised by all state taxes combined in that year (U.S. Bureau of the Census 1989). So even before adding in the cost of extending coverage to the uninsured, merely shifting what is now financed through private insurance into the public sector would require, on average, a more than 50 percent increase in the size of state government budgets. To the extent that financing is merely shifted, wages and profits would rise in some combination to offset the tax increase, *on average,* but individual businesses and workers are understandably wary of how such an enormous shift would affect them. In addition, providers of medical services tend not to look favorably on the idea of concentrating so much buying power into government hands. The health insurance industry worries about what role would be left for it to play in such a revamped system.

A natural alternative is to build on the current employment-based insurance system, requiring or encouraging more employers to provide coverage for their workers, and adding a "safety net" public program or set of programs to accommodate the remaining uninsured. Such an approach is surely less threatening to providers and to health insurers, and at least at first glance it appears that it might be accomplished with little expansion of state government budgets. Numerous studies have shown that as many as three-quarters of the current uninsured are in

77

households with at least one worker (Brown 1989). If employers could be induced to cover most of that group, so it is hoped, picking up the remainder with public coverage might be manageable.

What would seem to be the main virtue of this approach—the fact that it is an incremental change that builds from the system already in place—may, however, be its fatal flaw. By extending insurance coverage to all, it would boost substantially the demand for medical care in a system that already is ineffective in controlling the rate of increase of costs.[1] It would be administratively simpler to *implement* than a single state insurance plan (because it would rely on existing institutions), but over the long run it would not reduce the enormous administrative costs of the system in the way that a move to a single plan could (Himmelstein and Woolhandler 1989). In fact, by causing many more two-earner households to get coverage for each earner, it would create additional problems of coordination of benefits and probably add overhead cost to the system.

Universal coverage by this route is also likely to require higher state expenditures than it first appears. Most of the uninsured do indeed have some connection to the workforce, but the working uninsured tend to earn quite low wages or be employed only part time or part of the year. Employers will be very reluctant to bear the cost of insuring them. It is also true that many poor individuals and families who are now counted as insured pay for their own nongroup coverage out-of-pocket or must pay the full premiums to receive coverage from employers. With a public safety net available, many of them could drop their current insurance and move to subsidized public coverage. Employers who now cover their workers only reluctantly might also find it advantageous to drop coverage and turn their employees over to the public sector. These possibilities are explored quantitatively later in this chapter, using data from Michigan.

Expanding Private Coverage

Proponents of this approach to universal coverage see private insurance at the center, expanding its current role, with the state ready to support those who would remain uncovered. It is therefore appropriate to focus the discussion first on the steps that would be taken to expand employment-based coverage, as these will determine the size and composition of the population left to be covered publicly. There is a broad range of possibilities as to who among the current uninsured would be affected by a mandate directed at employers. Employers might be required by law to provide coverage to their employees, or they might be given an option of paying a special tax instead. Coverage of dependents might or might not be required. Exemptions or special rules might apply to some types of workers (e.g., part-time or seasonal employees) or types of firms (small or new businesses).

Approaches Implemented or Proposed

We can gain a sense of the range of options being considered by looking at several routes to expanding employer coverage already implemented or proposed. Hawaii is the one state with real experience; it has had mandated health insurance since the passage of its Prepaid Health Care Act in 1974 (American Hospital Association 1988). Employers there must provide health insurance for those workers who have completed at least four consecutive weeks of work, are working at least 20 hours per week, and whose monthly wage is at least 86.67 times the minimum hourly. Employees are only obligated to contribute 1.5 percent of gross wages toward the premium. The employer must offer dependent coverage, but is not required to pay for it. Some groups are exempted, including government employees, seasonal farm workers, and workers in family-owned businesses.

Massachusetts has gained much notoriety as the second state to legislate an expansion of employer-provided insurance (Enthoven and Kronick 1989). It seeks to induce coverage by taxing firms that do not provide it at 12 percent of wages, up to $1,680 per employee. The tax is not scheduled to take effect until 1992, so no experience with it yet exists. Employers with five or fewer employees, temporary or seasonal employees, and employees working less than 20 hours per week are all to be excluded. Employees with insurance coverage from some other source may also decline coverage, and the employer need not pay a tax.

Some proposals for mandating coverage at the federal level have also been widely discussed. One is the Basic Health Benefits for All Americans Act, introduced in Congress by Senator Kennedy and Representative Waxman. It would require that employers provide coverage for employees working at least 17.5 hours per week, as well as for dependents if they are not covered elsewhere. Employed dependents could retain coverage through their parents' plans. Employers would be required to pay 80 percent of the premium for employees working at least 25 hours per week and a smaller share for those working between 17.5 and 24 hours. A federal subsidy to small businesses for costs in excess of 5 percent of gross revenues is also included.

Another proposal is the "Consumer-Choice Health Plan for the 1990s" (Enthoven and Kronick 1989).[2] Under it, employers would be required to cover all employees working at least 25 hours per week, along with their dependents not otherwise covered. For part-time and seasonal employees, the employer could instead pay a tax of 8 percent of wages up to $1,800 per worker. For small businesses, payments for health benefits would be capped at 8 percent of total payroll.

Issues Surrounding Expanded Private Coverage

The similarities and differences among these approaches provide some food for thought for states interested in expanding employer-provided coverage.

1. *Legal Mandate or Tax Incentives?* The federal proposals and the Hawaii law *require* that employers provide coverage, at least for full-time workers. This may not be an option for a state at this time; in fact, it violates the Employee Retirement Income Security Act (ERISA). When the Hawaii law was tested in court, it was ruled to be preempted by ERISA, although a later amendment to ERISA made an exception for the Hawaii case. In the current climate of strong business opposition to mandated benefits,[3] further exceptions seem unlikely.

The alternative to a direct mandate is a so-called "play or pay" tax, to which firms not providing health insurance benefits are subject, as in Massachusetts.[4] Even apart from the legal difficulties with mandating, this approach has certain advantages. In principle, the tax can be set high enough that nearly all firms will provide coverage rather than pay it, so it does not necessarily lead to fewer individuals gaining coverage. At the same time, it preserves an element of choice for the employer.

More important, mandating almost of necessity involves exceptions. Employers of low-wage workers employed only a few hours a week cannot be expected to guarantee health insurance coverage, nor, perhaps, can a small start-up business not yet proven financially viable. But making exceptions means drawing lines, raising questions of fairness between similar cases that fall on opposite sides of the division. Furthermore, business decisions are distorted by the presence of these exceptions. If health insurance coverage need not be provided to those working less than, say, 20 hours per week, 25-hour employees may be shifted to 18 hours. If firms with five or fewer employees are exempt, decisions about expanding (or contracting) will be influenced by this fact.

Use of the tax may eliminate the need for all or at least most exceptions. While employers of part-time or very low-wage workers should not be expected to make the same contribution to health insurance coverage as others, they can be required to contribute in proportion to wages paid. This seems more fair than exempting some types of workers entirely, it reduces certain labor market distortions, and it provides a source of revenue for partially financing the coverage of those who will not get insurance through their employers. In the remainder of this discussion, I assume that coverage is not to be legally mandated, but rather induced through the use of a tax.

2. *What Must the Employer Do to Avoid the Tax?* One possibility is that employers are given a credit, dollar-for-dollar against tax owed, for payments for health care coverage made on behalf of employees. The problem with this approach is that it gives no incentive to spend less on coverage than an employer's maximum total tax liability—a dollar saved on coverage just becomes an additional tax dollar owed. The employer's incentive for cost consciousness in purchasing insurance is thereby attenuated. In addition, it is desirable to set the tax liability rather high to discourage firms from opting out of providing coverage. The combination of a high tax liability and dollar-for-dollar credit could stimulate additional spending on health coverage for those who are already well insured, contributing further to growing health costs.

The alternative is to waive the tax if some specified share (80 percent is commonly suggested) of the premium for a "qualified plan" is paid by the employer, regardless of the cost to the employer. In that way, a dollar saved in purchasing coverage goes directly back to the firm, enhancing its incentive to buy wisely. This approach requires that a qualified plan be defined, and raises the possibility that much currently held coverage may be ruled inadequate. But if truly universal coverage for a basic set of services is the goal, it makes sense to require that employer-provided coverage meet certain criteria. Defining a qualified plan also provides an opportunity to assure that particular cost-containment features be included, if that is desired.

3. *Coverage of Dependents and Those Currently in Public Programs.* Except for the Hawaii case, in all of the examples discussed above employers who provide coverage must cover dependents of their employees. In light of the large number of current uninsured who are dependents (mainly children) of workers (see chapter 2 of this volume), such a requirement seems a natural element of this strategy for universal coverage. In fact, it is probably good policy to let workers who are dependent children of other workers get their coverage through their parents, rather than their own employers. Families would be kept together for insurance purposes, reducing administrative costs to at least some degree. More important, very young workers usually earn low wages and have high job turnover rates. Requiring their own employers to provide insurance or even pay a tax may be particularly burdensome, and may have adverse employment effects.

Some workers or dependents of workers may have insurance coverage from existing government programs, especially Medicare or Medicaid. Because federal funds contribute heavily to the finance of these programs (Medicare is entirely federally financed, Medicaid about half, with some variation across states), it is probably not in the interest of a state to encourage that this coverage be replaced by an employer. In particular, the requirement that employers provide coverage or pay a tax probably should not extend to employees 65 and over, who are almost always eligible for Medicare. Excluding the elderly may, however, lead to political problems or charges of inequity if the basic package of services available to all the nonelderly is perceived as more extensive than what Medicare offers.

4. Efforts to Expand Availability of Coverage. While the phenomenon of workers without insurance coverage is by no means limited to small businesses, it is well documented that small firms are much less likely to offer coverage than are larger ones. An important reason is that premium costs for similar coverage are much higher for small firms. Available evidence on the magnitude of the difference is sketchy, but a difference in cost of $40 per $100 of benefits between a firm with fewer than 10 employees and one with more than 100 employees is probably a conservative estimate (American Hospital Association 1988; Danzon 1989). These cost differences stem from higher administrative and marketing costs for insuring small firms, and from insurers' concerns about adverse selection.

A reduction in that cost differential would by itself increase the number of small businesses offering insurance. Without a reduction, even rather strong tax incentives might not be enough to induce provision by very many additional small firms. Most proposals for expanding private coverage therefore include attempts to enhance the availability of insurance and improve the terms upon which it is offered to small firms. One option is for the state to create a single large insurance pool, which might also contain those gaining public coverage. Firms could be permitted to buy into the pool on a community-rated basis (the same rates would be available for all firms within a particular area of the state), with different rates for individual, couple, and family coverage.

This approach, with one large pool encompassing most of the current uninsured, would be in essence a scaled-down version of a state insurance plan, with many of the attendant advantages and disadvantages. Marketing costs could be considerably reduced, at least some administrative economies could be realized, and if enrollment in the pool were large enough, problems of adverse selection would be minimized. Some firms would, in effect, subsidize others under such an arrangement, however. Each employer would pay premiums intended to reflect the costs of providing coverage to an "average" firm with a similar mix of workers by family type, but not all firms are average. Firms who employ workers at higher-than-average risk, due to age or other factors, would pay the same premiums as everyone else, and the extra costs of their coverage would be spread across all participants in the plan.

The implications for health care costs of having a single large pool are also very important to consider. While the pool concentrates the buying power of small firms and thereby gives them some clout in the market, it also blunts their individual incentive to use that power effectively. If a firm has only a single option for purchasing insurance (i.e., through the pool) at rates over which it has no control, the firm has no role to play in assuring that it receives good coverage at a reasonable cost. Incentives for cost control can of course be built into the benefit package, with copayments, deductibles, and so forth. To a large extent, however, the responsibility for controlling costs (and assuring quality) would fall on the administrators of the pool.

Alternatively, market competition can be relied on for cost control and quality assurance, along the lines suggested by Enthoven and Kronick (1989). Competing qualified insurance plans might be made available to small businesses, with a state agency serving as a broker, certifying which plans are qualified, providing information to firms to facilitate comparisons among plans, managing the enrollment process, and generally administering the rules of the game. The basic idea is that giving firms a choice provides a better opportunity to satisfy individual preferences, and promotes competition among insurers to hold down costs while maintaining high quality.

But the most thoughtful proponents of this approach recognize that *managing* competition is essential and by no means easy (Enthoven 1986, 1988). There are difficult questions regarding the dimensions along which insurers should be permitted to compete. On what bases, for example, should they be permitted to set different premiums for different firms? Given the opportunity, insurers will compete to attract firms with relatively healthy workers. The most obvious way to do so is to charge lower premiums to firms with younger, healthier workforces. If this is permitted, firms employing workers who are bad health risks (and in a firm with few employees it may only take one case of serious illness) may find no good options available to them. They will choose to let their employees turn to public coverage, which will become a dumping ground for those at highest risk.

Requiring insurers to community rate would not eliminate all these problems. If required to community rate, insurers might attempt to tailor the benefit packages they offer to be particularly attractive to the healthy, or in subtle ways make it difficult for the chronically ill to receive covered services. Firms of moderate size expecting their experience to be better than average would have an incentive to self-insure, if that is still an option.

An important but still unanswered question about the competitive approach favored by Enthoven and Kronick is whether sufficient numbers of insurers would be willing to come forward and comply with the rules of the game, so that the potential benefits of choice and competition could actually be achieved.

Likely Effects on Firms and Workers

Employer Responses to a "Play or Pay" Tax

If employers are given a choice of providing insurance or paying a tax, it is no simple matter to predict how many individuals would gain employer-provided coverage under any particular plan. Surely the firm would look at which option, tax or coverage, is cheaper from its point of view. But employers have an interest in keeping their workers happy, so they will also be influenced by what the worker prefers.[5] The employer will be less likely to provide insurance if good public coverage is available free to workers than if an uncovered worker faces a premium or tax for public coverage *in addition to* the employer's tax. Complicating the firm's problem is the fact that it cannot decide on an employee-by-employee basis whether to provide coverage or pay the tax, but rather must make blanket decisions that apply at least to broad groups of employees.[6] High-wage workers in predominantly low-wage firms may end up without insurance from their employers (because it is not worthwhile to cover the entire firm). The converse would also be true.

Unless the tax rate is set very high, however, it is likely that for many low-wage and part-time workers employers will find it cheaper to pay the tax rather than provide coverage. Suppose, for example, that the tax rate is 10 percent and a worker is employed 20 hours per week and earning $5 per hour. The tax owed would be $10 per week or about $40 per month, far less than the cost of insurance coverage, even for a single individual.

It is appealing to suppose that all firms already providing coverage would continue to do so when the additional tax inducement is added, but this is unlikely. In many cases, the current coverage may not meet the standards for a qualified plan, the employer may be paying less than the share of the premium required, or the employer may not be covering dependents. The public safety net could also provide a better alternative to employer group coverage than is currently available for most workers. For these reasons, at least some employers now paying a share of the costs of their employees' coverage would choose to drop coverage and pay the tax instead. Many workers now counted as having employer group coverage would thus move to public coverage under this sort of package.

Incidence of the Costs of New Coverage and Labor Market Effects

Who would bear the costs of new employer-provided coverage and how the package would affect labor markets depend on the interaction of a number of factors, including the nature of public coverage and the terms upon which it is made available to those not covered in the workplace. The analysis is pursued in more detail in chapter 8. As a first approximation, however, standard economics suggests that in the long run the money wages of those who gain coverage would fall by about the cost of coverage to the employer. This conclusion is based on two presumptions. First, firms make employment decisions on the basis of total compensation per worker (wages plus benefits); they will only choose to hire the same number of workers if compensation does not change. Second, the supply of workers (and work hours) will be about the same at either wage level. This simple analysis has very strong implications. It says that those who gain employer-provided coverage will, for the most part, pay for it themselves (in the form of lower wages), and that total labor costs, business profits, and prices will therefore be little affected.

These predictions may be substantially correct, but they need to be qualified in several important ways. First, the phrase "in the long run" deliberately sidesteps the issue of what happens right away. While some employers would cut wages if forced to add insurance, others may find it impossible or unwise to do so (for example, due to existing collective bargaining agreements). Their workers would get smaller wage *increases* than otherwise, until eventually the difference in wage level had compensated for the cost of insurance. In the meantime, however, those firms would suffer lower profits, would (to the extent possible) pass some of their higher costs into prices, and in some cases would not survive.

Second, the presumption that labor supply is unaffected by changes in wage rates and insurance coverage is not entirely accurate, particularly for two-earner couples. Empirical studies have shown that decisions about whether and how much to work by the lower-earning spouse are rather strongly influenced by the terms of compensation. Frequently, these secondary earners already have insurance through a spouse's job. Forcing their own employers to provide coverage (or pay a tax) will reduce the money wages the employers are willing to offer, and thereby reduce the workers' incentive to work. Employers will in turn find such secondary earners more difficult and expensive to hire.

The numbers of secondary earners affected in this way are quite large. Analyses of national proposals for mandated insurance coverage (Gordon 1988; Thorpe 1989) have suggested that, of all workers gaining insurance under a federal mandate, roughly half already have coverage through an employed family member.

Finally, for workers at or near the legal minimum wage, wages cannot be reduced enough to compensate for the added costs of coverage. If wages cannot be reduced at all, the cost of coverage (or the tax) is effectively an add-on to the minimum wage. For those close to the minimum wage, it is likely that most employers will find it cheaper to pay the tax than to provide coverage, and hence the tax rate becomes an upper bound on the extra increase in labor cost felt by the employer. Recent empirical studies have found that employment of minimum wage workers declines by about 1 to 3 percent in response to a 10 percent increase in the minimum wage (Brown 1988). A 10 percent payroll tax would have a similar effect.[7] A higher tax rate would induce more insurance coverage on behalf of low-wage workers, but it would also create more adverse employment effects while leading to higher prices and lower profits for those firms that employ such workers.

Costs of New Public Programs

No attempt to expand the reach of insurance in the workplace can by itself lead to universal coverage. Although most of the uninsured have some connection to the labor force, there are still large numbers who have none and who do not qualify for any existing public insurance program. A universal system needs a safety net program or set of programs to assure that they are covered. Those who have no proof of other insurance could be assessed (probably through the existing state tax system) an income-based premium. They might then be given Medicaid-style coverage, or placed in a new large insurance pool that also includes employees of small businesses. If a more competitive approach is desired, this population could be given vouchers and, where possible, allowed to choose among competing qualified plans. Issues of equity (as well as work incentives) could arise if the level of coverage guaranteed is perceived as less attractive than Medicaid.

As discussed at the outset, an obvious appeal of this route to universal coverage is that it requires a much smaller expansion of government budgets than would an entirely tax-financed system. The hope—not entirely without foundation—is that the additional commitment of state dollars required might be held to an acceptable magnitude. After all, most workers and their families already have coverage, and most of the uninsured are in households with at least one worker. If coverage could be extended further in the workplace, and no one lost coverage they now hold, a relatively small residual group might be left to be picked up in the public sector.

What becomes clear on a close examination of the data, however, is that depending on exactly how the total package is designed, large numbers of individuals who are currently insured could move to heavily subsidized public coverage. The key to seeing this point is to recognize that many individuals now have private coverage and are counted as insured, yet are quite poor. Thorpe (1989) has estimated that for the nation as a whole in 1987, 6.7 million individuals in poverty households had private insurance, as did an additional 4.5 million individuals in households under 125 percent of the poverty level. Some of them got group coverage through employers, but paid much or all of the cost themselves. Others purchased their own nongroup insurance. (Thorpe estimated that altogether about 10 million individuals had only such coverage.) Given their low incomes, it is likely that much of this coverage is quite limited and would not satisfy standards for a qualified plan. Unless the tax rate is set quite high, few in this group can be expected to gain employer-provided coverage, and many may lose the partial employer support that they now have. Depending again on the tax rate, others at incomes substantially above poverty may lose private coverage.

The split between private or public coverage might be largely a matter of indifference from a policy perspective if the taxes paid by employers plus supplemental taxes directly on individuals covered the costs of the newly publicly insured. But this too would not happen, even at quite high tax rates.

An Analysis of Michigan Data

These ideas may be illustrated with data from Michigan. For other states interested in this approach to universal coverage, the method of analysis may be of more interest than the quantitative results. I have estimated the net increase in public insurance coverage under the kind of package being discussed here, using data from the March 1988 Current Population Survey (CPS).[8] The details assumed for the package are as follows.

All employers must provide coverage to all employees, and spouses and dependents not otherwise covered, or pay a payroll tax. The only exceptions are that any workers who have coverage under an existing government program (Medicaid, Medicare, or CHAMPUS, a federal program for dependents of military personnel) need not be covered by the employer, and workers who are under 18 and living with parents or between 18 and 22 and students are to get coverage through their parents. Three tax rates are considered: 10, 15 and 20 percent. Presumably, a ceiling on the amount of tax owed per employee would be included in such a package. I do not specify one for my analysis, assuming instead that all workers above particular earnings levels would be provided coverage by their employers.

Those who are not already covered in a public program and do not get coverage from an employer or purchase it themselves are automatically participants in a new public insurance program. For that they are assessed a tax (which could be filed with the regular state income tax in states that have one) on all income above a $2,000 per person exemption, at a rate equal to that of the payroll tax, up to a point at which a fair premium has been paid. Any payroll tax already paid on an individual's behalf would be credited dollar-for-dollar against income tax owed. The self-employed would, as a result of this income tax, have the same responsibility in providing for their own insurance that employers have for employees.[9] This income tax (or income-based premium) places a rather heavy burden on the poor among the current uninsured. Despite this, we will see that it raises relatively little revenue.

To estimate who ends up with public coverage, the CPS sample of individuals must first be grouped into family units that would be kept together for insurance purposes. Each unit is classified as either already having public coverage, retaining or picking up private coverage, or (the residual) entering the new public program. In general, family units are put in the private insurance group if earnings are high enough (singly or in combination) that payroll taxes paid in 1988 would be at least as large as 80 percent of the estimated 1988 premium for a qualified plan. Workers who do not meet this test but already have employment-based coverage are assumed to keep it, if all members of the family unit have coverage and the employer pays at least part of the cost. This last assumption is optimistic, as surely some of those employers would drop coverage.[10]

The results of the analysis for Michigan, as reported in Table 1, show substantial enrollments in the new public program, both because many of the current uninsured fail to gain private coverage (even with tax rates as high as 20 percent), and because many of the insured shift over. According to the March 1988 CPS, the total number of uninsured under age 65 in Michigan is about 870,000.[11] The estimated enrollment in the new program ranges from 1.2 million with a 10 percent tax to 770,000 if the tax is 20 percent. At the lower rate, only about 200,000 of the state's uninsured gain employment-based coverage, while about 490,000 of the insured move to public coverage. At the 20 percent rate, about 520,000 of the uninsured would gain coverage from employers, but about two-thirds of that number (320,000) would be leaving their current coverage to enter the public program.

Table 1
Numbers Gaining Public Coverage (100,000s)
Illustration for Michigan

	Tax rate		
	10 percent	15 percent	20 percent
Total	11.7	9.5	7.7
Number already insured	4.9	4.0	3.2

SOURCES: March 1988 CPS for Michigan and author's assumptions about participation.

Table 2 shows the expected age composition of the public program at each of the tax rates, along with comparative data on the composition of the Michigan population under age 65 and the Michigan uninsured population. The composition of the group does not change much as the tax rate changes, but it does look rather different from the current uninsured population. In particular, those aged 15 to 20 or over 44 would form a considerably larger share of the new program enrollments than they do of the current uninsured population. Both subgroups contain relatively large numbers of insured individuals who would find public coverage an attractive alternative. In the younger subgroup, many are 18 to 20 years of age and not in school, but apparently covered under parents' policies. The size of the public program could be kept down to some degree by broadening the definition of dependent and requiring that some of these individuals continue to be covered through their parents. Table 2 also shows that a relatively large share of uninsured males aged 26 to 44 would gain employment-based insurance and therefore not require public coverage.

Table 2

Composition of the New Public Program (Percent by Age Group)
Illustration for Michigan

Age group	Tax rate			Population under 65	Current uninsured
	10 percent	15 percent	20 percent		
0-4	8.2	8.8	8.9	7.8	10.6
5-14	12.7	13.1	12.1	15.2	18.3
15-20	15.4	15.8	15.0	10.8	8.4
21-25	16.8	16.6	17.6	10.6	17.7
26-44 (Male)	13.1	12.3	11.7	17.0	21.9
26-44 (Female)	12.1	10.9	10.3	16.7	10.5
45-64	21.7	22.5	24.5	21.9	12.6

SOURCES: March 1988 CPS for Michigan and author's assumptions about participation.

Gross costs for the new public program under different assumptions about its size and the benefit package are reported in Table 3. The cost numbers are based on my calculations using data from Blue Cross-Blue Shield of Michigan in its Area Rated Groups line of business, sold mainly to small firms. The Basic Package is traditional Blue Cross-Blue Shield coverage, covering mainly inpatient hospital care and associated professional services. The Expanded Package adds major medical coverage of a broader set of services with deductible and copayment provisions, as well as coverage of prescription drugs with low copayments. Some advantages of these numbers are that they are based on actual cost experience, not premiums, and were available by age category. Using them does not imply that public coverage would have to be of this type.

Table 3
Gross and Net Costs of the New Public Program ($100 millions)
Illustration for Michigan

	Tax rate		
	10 percent	**15 percent**	**20 percent**
Gross Cost			
Basic Package	10.6	8.6	7.2
Expanded Package	13.4	10.8	9.1
Revenue			
Payroll Tax	4.3	3.7	2.8
Income Tax	0.7	1.0	1.2
Net Cost			
Basic Package	5.5	3.9	3.3
Expanded Package	8.3	6.2	5.1

SOURCES: Author's calculations from March 1988 CPS for Michigan and Blue Cross-Blue Shield of Michigan 1988 cost experience for Area Rated Groups line of business.

Costs amount to a little more than $900 per enrollee per year for the Basic Package, and about $1,150 for the Expanded Package (in both cases, a little higher for the population mix at the 20 percent tax rate). If other estimates are available and believed more appropriate, they could of course be easily substituted. See chapter 6 for additional discussion of costs of coverage and their relationship to the benefit package offered.

Table 3 also includes estimates of tax revenues the entire program package would generate, and then nets these out against gross program costs. Payroll tax revenues fall as the tax rate increases, as substantially more firms choose to provide coverage rather than pay the tax. Income tax revenues increase with the tax rate, but still amount to only about $150 per year per enrollee at the high 20 percent rate. Most of those who end up in the public program under this tax rate are quite poor, and frequently they would have no income tax liability due to payroll taxes already paid on their behalf.

The bottom line net costs to state government (in 1989 dollars) range from about $330 million with the Basic Package and 20 percent tax rate to about $830 million with the Expanded Package and 10 percent rate. These figures are after netting out payroll tax and extra income tax revenues the program would generate. Universal coverage is not cheap. To put the numbers in some perspective, each $100 million would amount to about $12 for each Michigan resident under age 65, or would require adding roughly 0.13 percent to the state's broad-based income tax, currently at 4.6 percent.

The experience in other states would of course be different, but not necessarily more favorable. The Medicaid program already covers a larger share of Michigan's poor population than is the case in most states. The share of the state's under-65 population without insurance is well below the national average. Based on 1986 and 1987 CPS numbers, the national share was over 17 percent compared with about 12 percent in Michigan.

Concluding Comments

The net costs to state government of taking this path to universal coverage, as identified in the previous section, do not all represent a net increase in medical services provided in the state. It is very likely that, with better financial access to medical care, the previously uninsured will consume more medical services than they currently do. But they use some care now, and pay some of the cost of it out of their own pockets. Much of that cost—for the uninsured who are poor—

would be shifted to the public sector. The same is true for those poor families now paying for their own insurance but who would switch to public coverage. Thus a share of the added costs to state government would really represent a shift from the uninsured and other poor families to the general taxpayer.

Much of the care currently received by the uninsured is also paid for in other less explicit ways, by providers accepting lower returns than they otherwise would, and by other payers paying more for the care received, to help cover the costs of care given to those who cannot pay. If state and local governments are already making payments for such uncompensated care, these could be folded into the new program and would reduce the amount of new revenue to be raised. To the extent that employers are now paying for uncompensated care, a system of universal coverage should bring downward pressure on the cost of employer-provided insurance. However, how the gains from a significant reduction in uncompensated care would be distributed among providers and various payers is not well understood.

Getting to universal coverage by expanding and supplementing the employment-based insurance system would not be easy, and would very likely require a significant increase in a state government's budget. No state should embark on this path unless it is willing to face that fact. But given a strong commitment to coverage for all, the necessary budget increase is not entirely outside the range of plausibility, and it is certainly far smaller than what would be needed for a Canadian model state health plan.

The costs of financing a combined public-private system at the point of implementation are surely an important factor affecting its political feasibility. What is probably more important, however, for the long-run success of such an approach is whether it can be implemented in a way that promotes a better balance between cost and quality improvements in health care, or whether it would merely add to already formidable pressures for ever-increasing costs.

NOTES

1. See the comments of Johnston on the proposal by the National Leadership Commission on Health Care (Johnston and Reinhardt 1989).

2. Viewing the Enthoven-Kronick proposal as merely a way of achieving universal insurance coverage does not do justice to the plan. It includes provisions (including a restructuring of existing tax subsidies for employer-provided insurance) aimed at harnessing market forces to promote cost containment and quality assurance in health care.

3. A recent survey of the membership of the National Association of Manufactures (Higgins and Co. 1989) found that 84 percent opposed mandated employer-provided health insurance, despite the fact that over 99 percent of the respondents were already providing health insurance benefits to their employees.

4. A national proposal by the National Leadership Commission on Health Care (1989) also has this feature.

5. Clearly this is true when workers are unionized, but even if not, it is in the firm's interest to provide a compensation package that is of most value to the worker for a given level of cost.

6. In the current environment, insurers usually insist on this to guard against the possibility that only bad health risks will choose to take coverage. Under the kind of program being discussed, the state would not want to permit individualized decisions for fear that bad risks would be pushed into public coverage to keep the employer's private insurance costs low.

7. It should be noted, however, that there would be no adverse employment effects for very young low-wage workers if they are expected to get insurance coverage through their parents.

8. Earnings and income figures in the March 1988 CPS are for 1987. I have updated them roughly to 1989 by increasing them by 6 percent. Estimates of the cost of coverage are also updated to 1989.

9. In this quantitative analysis, taxes paid by the self-employed with sufficiently high incomes are counted as part of payroll taxes.

10. In more detail, the classification scheme works as follows. A family unit *does not* enter the new public program if it is: (a) a single individual in an existing public program, or with earnings sufficient to pay $800 annually in payroll tax, or with group health already in his or her own name, for which an employer bears at least part of the cost; (b) a two-adult couple in which one member has earnings sufficient to pay $1,600 annually in payroll tax, or each individually meets the conditions in (a); (c) a family with children in which the head or spouse has earnings sufficient to pay $2,000 annually in payroll tax, or all members are currently covered, either by public programs or group health (for which an employer of the head or spouse pays at least part of the cost), or all but the head or spouse are covered by public programs and the remaining individual meets the conditions in (a).

11. This number is a good deal lower than that obtained from other recent waves of the CPS and may be an underestimate. See discussion by Moyer (1989) and Swartz and Purcell (1989).

References

American Hospital Association. 1988. *Promoting Health Insurance in the Workplace.* Chicago: American Hospital Association.

Brown, Charles. 1988. "Minimum Wage Laws: Are They Overrated?" *Journal of Economic Perspectives* 2 (Summer): 133-45.

Brown, E. Richard. 1989. "Access to Health Insurance in the United States," *Medical Care Review* 46 (Winter): 350-85.

Danzon, Patricia M. 1989. "Mandated Employment-Based Health Insurance: Incidence and Efficiency Effects." Unpublished paper.

Enthoven, Alain. 1986. "Managed Competition in Health Care and the Unfinished Agenda," *Health Care Financing Review* (supplement): 105-19.

_____. 1988. "Managed Competition: An Agenda for Action," *Health Affairs* 7 (Summer): 25-47.

_____ and Richard Kronick. 1989. "A Consumer-Choice Health Plan for the 1990s," *New England Journal of Medicine* 320 (January 5): 29-37 and (January 12): 94-101.

Gordon, Nancy M. 1988. Statement to the Subcommittee on Health and the Environment, Committee on Energy and Commerce, U.S. House of Representatives (April 15).

Higgins, A. Foster and Co. 1989. *National Association of Manufacturers Health Care Survey* (May).

Himmelstein, David U. and Steffie Woolhandler. 1989. "A National Health Program for the United States," *New England Journal of Medicine* 320 (January 12): 102-108.

Johnston, J. Bruce and Uwe E. Reinhardt. 1989. "Addressing the Health of a Nation: Two Views," *Health Affairs* 8 (Summer): 5-23.

Letsch, Suzanne W., Katharine R. Levit and Daniel R. Waldo. 1988. "National Health Expenditures, 1987," *Health Care Financing Review* 10 (Winter): 109-22.

Moyer, M. Eugene. 1989. "A Revised Look at the Number of Uninsured Americans," *Health Affairs* 8 (Summer): 102-10.

National Leadership Commission on Health Care. 1989. *For the Health of a Nation.*

Swartz, Katherine and Patrick J. Purcell. 1989. "Counting Uninsured Americans," *Health Affairs* 8 (Winter): 193-96.

Thorpe, Kenneth E. 1989. "Costs and Distributional Impacts of Employer Health Insurance Mandates and Medicaid Expansion," *Inquiry* 26 (Fall): 335-44.

U.S. Bureau of the Census. 1989. *State Tax Collections in 1988,* Series GF-88-1. Washington, DC: Government Printing Office.

5.1
Piecemeal Programs of Health Insurance for the Uninsured

Andrew J. Hogan
Michigan State University

The financing mechanisms of the U.S. health care system have developed in a piecemeal fashion over the last five decades to meet the needs of particular groups whose access to health care has differed significantly from the rest of the population at some point in time. These piecemeal programs are supplemented by individually purchased (nongroup) health insurance coverage. There is also a growing number of "free-riders" who do not maintain any insurance coverage and who lack the financial resources to meet the expenses of a serious illness. These uninsured "free-riders" account for a significant proportion of the uncompensated care hospitals are required to provide under emergency conditions.

This combination of piecemeal programs, nongroup coverage, and free-riding has, over the years, created a paradoxical stability for the current financing system, even as it appears to be spiraling toward collapse. Proposals such as those reviewed in the previous chapter face an enormous financial inefficiency, in that to increase health care spending for the uninsured by $1, current financing of $3 to $7 must be reorganized. For example, Needleman, et al. (1989) estimated that to increase spending for the uninsured in Pennsylvania by $393M, expenditures by employers would need to be increased by $779M, from individual insurance by $152M, from medicaid by $142M, with decreasing contributions by household out-of-pocket (–$334), charity care (–$189M), Medicare (–$74) and other government payments (–$82M). In total, $1,751M of health care spending has to be reorganized to increase spending for the uninsured by $393M, or $4.5 reorganized for each $1 of incremental spending. In a similar vein, Thorpe and Siegel (1989) estimate sizable differences in public and private costs when a

99

Medicaid expansion, a Medicaid Buy-In, and an employer-mandated approach are considered for adoption in different combinations.

Further piecemeal adjustments to the current system are significantly more manageable than large-scale reforms, politically if not financially. It may be that such piecemeal reforms can only postpone an inevitable collapse of the current system and the necessity of a large-scale reform or an overtly two-tiered system. A state not able or willing to undertake a major reform, however, might analyze its health care financing system to identify the major points of destabilization: the working poor, children, nonworking adults, high-risk individuals, providers of uncompensated care. The state could then implement a program to minimize the destablization of those critical points. Such piecemeal measures might actually stabilize a state health care system, at least for a time.

One area where special needs may exist is in the employed single-parent household. In Michigan, almost one-third of the uninsured children live with employed single parents. These uninsured single-parent families tend to have lower incomes than full families. Single parents are faced with a choice of an individual or a full-family (two-parent) health insurance policy, which is often actuarially unfair to the single-parent family and often involves unaffordaly high premiums. A piecemeal approach to lower the cost of health insurance to single-parent families is to mandate that insurers offer a single-parent policy. Such a mandate should require little administrative effort beyond the normal insurance commission monitoring of policies. The State of Michigan Employees Health Plan offers a parent-child option with premiums less than those for the two (dual) adult option and only 60 percent of the full-family premium.

Before undertaking any of the programs described in the rest of this chapter, a state should consider using all existing programs to their fullest extent, especially the Medicaid expansion for children, pregnant women, and the working poor. Some of the Medicaid expansions enacted during the 1980s include (National Health Policy Forum 1989):

- Deficit Reduction Act of 1984: coverage of children under age 5 where family income falls below AFDC eligibility thresholds; coverage of pregnant women who would become eligible if their children were born, and pregnant women who would qualify for the AFDC unemployed spouse program if the state were to offer it; automatic eligibility for infants born to Medicaid-eligible mothers.

- Consolidated Omnibus Budget Reconciliation Act of 1985: coverage of pregnant women with family incomes below state AFDC standards, even if not receiving AFDC, AFDC (unemployed), or SSI; 60 days of post-partum coverage for women eligible for Medicaid solely due to pregnancy; option to enhance the benefit package for pregnant women; extended coverage for adopted children with special health needs; sanctioned use of Medicaid case-management services.
- Omnibus Budget Reconciliation Act of 1986: extended coverage to pregnant women, children under 5 years, aged and disabled with incomes below 100 percent of poverty line; use of "presumptive eligibility" where designated prenatal care providers can screen and qualify pregnant women for temporary Medicaid coverage immediately.
- Omnibus Budget Reconciliation Act of 1987: permitted coverage of pregnant women and infants (< 1 year) in families with incomes below 185 percent of the federal poverty line; permitted coverage of all children under 8 years below poverty line.
- Medicare Catastrophic Coverage Act of 1988: mandatory coverage of pregnant women and children under 1 year with incomes below the poverty line.
- Family Support Act of 1988: mandatory continuation of Medicaid coverage for next 12 months for families receiving AFDC in three of previous six months; mandatory AFDC unemployed spouse program.

Some proportion of the uninsured population can be reduced by full implementation of all of these Medicaid expansions and aggressive outreach to find eligibles not currently participating. The remaining sections of this chapter will discuss the major options available to states that are willing and able to do more without undertaking large-scale reform: small employer pools, Medicaid Buy-In programs, high-risk pools, and uncompensated care programs.

Bibliography

National Health Policy Forum. 1989. ''Stretching the Limits of Medicaid for the Poor, Providers, and Private Payers: Are We Prepared to Pay the Price.'' Issue Brief No. 521. Washington, DC: George Washington University.

Needleman, J., J. Arnold, J. Sheils, L.S. Lewin. 1989. ''Meeting the Needs of the Uninsured and Underinsured Through Insurance Mandates and Direct Funding of Services: Lessons from National and State Analysis.'' Presented at the annual meeting of the Association for Health Services Research, Chicago.

Thorpe, K.E. and J.E. Siegel. 1989. ''Covering the Uninsured: Interactions Among Public and Private Sector Strategies,'' *JAMA* 262(15): 2114-2118.

5.2
Small Employer
Health Insurance Pools

Andrew J. Hogan
Stephen A. Woodbury
Michigan State University

Need for Small Employer Health Insurance Pools

Characteristics of Uninsured
and Underinsured Employees

Almost 60 percent of nonelderly adults without health insurance are employed (Swartz 1989). Almost half of these employed uninsured adults live in families with less than 200 percent of poverty income, and nearly two-thirds of them are employed by small firms, generally earning low wages (Moyer 1989).

The Health Insurance Survey of Michigan (Figure 1) indicates that less than half of all employees of small firms (fewer than 100 employees) have adequate health insurance coverage. About 20 percent are underinsured, in that physician's office visits are not covered or as evidenced by problems with inadequate coverage in the past year. Another 25 percent have adequate insurance but are only marginally insured, in that they have either nongroup coverage purchased with after-tax income or their employers make no contribution toward their premium. Ten percent of employees of small firms have coverage that is both marginal and inadequate.

Employed persons with nongroup coverage are likely to relinquish that coverage when small employer pool group coverage is offered. Firms offering poor health benefit coverage may replace it with coverage offered by the pool. Further, many employees in small firms, who are currently covered under a spouse's health plan, may decide to switch to coverage in their own name through their employer from the pool.

Figure 1
Adequacy of Health Insurance Coverage
by Firm Size

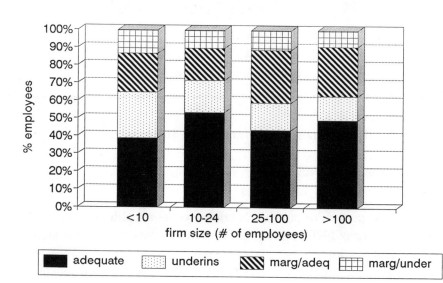

Source: Health Insurance Survey of Michigan

Key

adequate: good coverage with significant employer contribution.

underins: underinsured, physician office visits not covered, or problems encountered during last year.

marg/adeq: good coverage, with no employer contribution or nongroup coverage.

marg/under: underinsured, with no employer contribution or nongroup coverage.

Characteristics of Small Employer
Health Insurance Market

A recent survey of Michigan insurance carriers revealed that small employers ($<$100 FTEs) may pay premiums from 10 percent to 40 percent higher than the 500+ FTE firm for equivalent coverage (Health Management Associates 1989). Interestingly, the employees of small firms tend to be younger (and perhaps healthier) than their medium- and large-firm counterparts (Hogan 1989), which could make small employer health insurance premiums even more actuarially unfair than the simple premium differential might indicate.

As health insurance premiums have become increasingly less affordable, both small firms and insurance carriers have developed strategies to avoid the risk of paying for adverse selection. In the small firm, one significant illness can lead to a very adverse loss ratio for the carrier. Carriers will attempt to avoid this risk prospectively by various underwriting approaches: exclusion of pre-existing conditions, exclusion of employees with pre-existing conditions or even termination of the policy once serious conditions are identified.

Carriers not adopting these strategies would soon find themselves inundated by demand from excluded firms. The resulting adverse selection will quickly cause unfavorable loss ratios, leading to rising premiums. If the premiums are community-rated, then there will be a flight of small firms without significant risks to those carriers offering lower premiums with restrictive underwriting practices.

Over the years these strategies have led to an enormous churning in the small employer health insurance market. Small employers change carriers readily, and carriers selling to small employers offer limited products which are heavily underwritten and whose premiums often escalate quickly after a year or two. Many large carriers have abandoned the small employer market altogether. Larger employers have also abandoned the health insurance market to avoid sharing the risk of adverse selection and are now almost always under some kind of experience-rated or self-funded arrangement (Gabel et al. 1989). In summary, the employment-based health insurance market has come to rest primarily on small and medium employers purchasing from small and medium carriers, all of whom have as a major strategy the management of adverse selection. In some states, such as Michigan, Blue Cross-Blue Shield plans are required to act as insurers of last resort and to insure a significant number of small firms.

The high level of carrier-client churning has contributed to the high administrative costs in the small employer health insurance market. As turbulent as the small employer health insurance market is, it is not surprising that small employers have not organized themselves well to deal with one of the major forces in the health care financing in the 1980s: cost-shifting. In the early 1980s, federal and state governments began enacting legislation and administrative rules to limit their liability for health care cost inflation; this came after a decade of unsuccessful attempts to contain health care costs. The Medicare and Medicaid programs changed their reimbursement policies from cost-plus to fixed fees. After years of budgetary restraint, these fees are now significantly below those paid by private insurers (Thorpe, Siegel, Dailey 1989). Whether these fees have fallen below the cost of care is a matter of some dispute. However, once the separation was made between costs and payments for two large payers, other payers began to follow suit. Large employers have been able to leverage their size either with carriers and third-party administrators or through group purchasing arrangements to gain preferential treatment. The result has been that large employer premiums have been increasing at one-half the rate of small employer premiums (Kramon 1989). Small employers have been unable to defend their interests in this process of cost-shifting.

Rationale for Small Employer Health Insurance Pool

The pool attempts to give small employers some of the advantages that large employers enjoy in the health insurance market: elimination of underwriting and exclusions, an organized response to cost-shifting and premium differentials, and an improved benefit design. By joining together, small employers can create a self-funded multiple employer welfare trust that should, over time, bring their health benefit expenses in line with actual costs. Such a self-funded plan can resist cost-shifting and will provide a reasonably stable source of insurance coverage for small employers.

The major challenge for such a pool is the large number of "high-risk" individuals purchasing group or nongroup coverage who will rush into the pool if premiums are set at a level to entice "good risk" small employers not currently offering benefits to join. Adverse selection problems could be severe, and the small employer program could easily become a "high-risk" pool. In addition to adverse selection, the small employer pool will need to contend with the high level of employee turnover and financial instability of small firms (Health Management Associates 1989; Brown 1989). For these reasons, some public subsidy will be required to offset the costs of the high-risk individuals who will join the pool in disproportionate numbers.

Given the large number of small firms currently offering benefits who are either paying a high percent of payroll for the benefit or who are purchasing an inferior benefit, a small employer pool is likely, upon offering a reasonably priced plan, to be inundated by small employers who currently offer benefits and who qualify for subsidies. Such a program could spend substantial subsidies and not appreciably affect the number of uninsured individuals. A major policy consideration is the suggestion that the small employer pool be open only to employers who do not currently offer health benefits. In the long run, excluding employers who currently offer health benefits from participation in the program is probably unfair, but the approach may be workable as a transitional measure.[1]

An additional policy issue is whether an employee must work some minimum number of hours per week to qualify for health insurance. Other things being equal, participation of part-time workers increases premium costs more than it increases payroll, resulting in more subsidy payments if premiums are to be affordable.

Administration of Small Employer Health Insurance Programs

One approach is the creation of a small business health insurance pool open to all businesses with less than 25 employees, new businesses (< 1 year) with less than 100 employees, and the self-employed. The state insurance bureau could annually determine actuarially fair premiums plus administrative loadings for the small business pool. Premiums should not be experience-rated to encourage coverage for high-risk employees, if subsidies can be obtained.

To make the purchase of health insurance more attractive to the small employer, premiums can be subsidized as a percent of total payroll. Eligible employers would pay full premiums as long as the total health benefit expense is less than, for example, 4 percent of payroll. Employers would pay 50 percent of the total premiums in excess of 4 percent but less than 8 percent of payroll, and they would pay 10 percent of total premiums in excess of 8 percent of payroll. To reduce free-riding, at least 75 percent of a firm's uninsured workers would have to be covered for a firm to receive such a subsidy. Employers providing evidence of financial distress could be allowed to delay or reduce premium payments up to one year. Employers may require employees to share in the payment of premiums, as long as the employee earns at least 125 percent of the federal minimum wage.[2] Employer premium contributions must at least equal employee premium contributions for the firm to receive a premium subsidy.

An alternative subsidy mechanism is to make subsidy payments directly to employees and to base the amount of the subsidy on the economic status of the employee and his or her dependents. Employees with household incomes less than 200 percent of poverty would receive premium subsidies to supplement their own or their employer's premium contributions. Eligible employers could pay full premiums for all employees whose family income exceeds 200 percent of poverty income. For those between 100 and 200 percent of poverty:

$$\text{Premium share} = \frac{\text{Adjusted family income}}{\text{Poverty rate income}} - 1.$$

A somewhat more modest alternative approach is to extend the Health Care Access Project (HCAP) being undertaken in Genesee and Marquette Counties in the State of Michigan (Smith 1989). The HCAP program is one of 15 Robert Wood Johnson access demonstration projects. The program is open to employers who do not now offer health benefits and it uses existing insurance mechanisms (usually the local Chamber of Commerce area-rated group plans offered by Blue Cross-Blue Shield of Michigan). HCAP subsidizes up to one-third of the total premium contribution for eligible establishments. HCAP will further subsidize some or all of the employee premium contribution based on family income.

In spite of fairly generous premium subsidies, HCAP and other access demonstration projects have been able to enroll only about 20 percent of eligible employers contacted (Perry 1989). The chief advantages of the HCAP-type approach are their reliance on existing insurance programs and the easily understood one-third subsidy. Subsidies based on health benefit expense as a percent of payroll or on family income better target the subsidy dollar and will probably produce higher participation in the long run, but will be harder to understand and more expensive to administer in the short run.

Benefit Options

Selection of a small employer pool benefit package is, by necessity, market driven. The package must be acceptable to those who buy it, but it must not be so rich that it creates more health care cost inflation by causing the coverage offered by firms currently providing benefits to expand. Thus, the package selected is slightly below that typically offered by small employers.

Two possible benefit packages can be considered: a full benefit plan and a plan covering only outpatient services. Either policy offered by the insurance pool should cover employees and dependents. The full health insurance policy offered by the pool would cover inpatient hospital room and board, surgical care, diagnostic x-ray and laboratory, and emergency room care. Both plans will cover outpatient diagnostic and preventive services, laboratory and x-ray, physician office visits, prescription drugs and home health care. The plans should have modest deductibles and copayments for most services to maintain utilization within the financial means of low-income employees.

NOTES

1. Under the Robert Wood Johnson-financed Health Care Access project (HCAP) demonstration in the Michigan counties of Genesee and Marquette, there is no incentive for an employer to drop current coverage in order to qualify for participation in the program because of the limited time frame of the demonstration and the uncertainties about the future. With a permanent program, an employer could more reasonably choose to drop health insurance in the short run to receive the long-term subsidies offered by the program.

2. Employee premium contributions are not an effective cost-containment measure when there is only one plan to choose and should be used sparingly with poverty groups. Copayments and deductibles are more effective in limiting excessive health care utilization, but again the low-income levels of many of the uninsured make reliance on these cost-containment mechanisms onerous.

Appendix to Chapter 5.2

Small Employer Pool Percent of Payroll Subsidy

Figure A.1 illustrates how the premium subsidy mechanism will work. Suppose a small employer has one employee earning $1,000 per month in total compensation, $100 of which is used to pay for health insurance. The first 4 percent of gross payroll ($40) is paid by the workplace (employer and employee may share this expense). The next 4 percent of payroll (from 4 percent to 8 percent) is divided evenly between the workplace and the subsidy, $20 each. The last 2 percent of payroll (8 percent to 10 percent) is paid 90 percent by the subsidy ($18) and 10 percent by the workplace ($2). The workplace expense is then $40 + $20 + $2 = $62. The subsidy expense is $0 + $20 + $18 = $38. If the worker were to earn only $500, the subsidy would grow to $0 + $10 + $54 = $64. If the worker earns $2,000/month, the subsidy would fall to $0 + $10 + $0 = $10.

Small Employer Pool Family Income Subsidy

All employees of small employers participating in the pool can apply for premium subsidies. For employees with incomes less than 200 percent of poverty, subsidies will be provided, as is illustrated in Figure A.2.

Figure A1
Employer/Employee Premium Contributions
(Small Employer Pool)

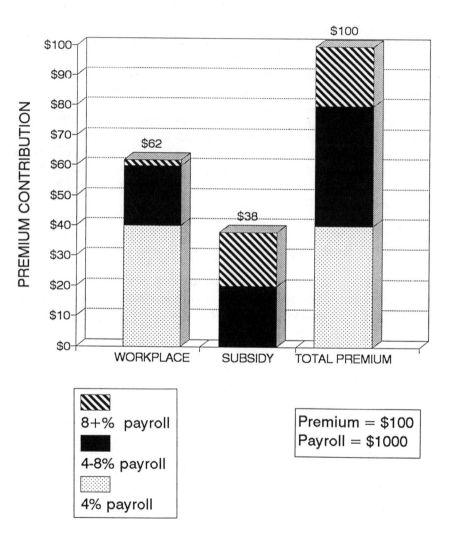

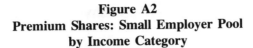

Figure A2
Premium Shares: Small Employer Pool
by Income Category

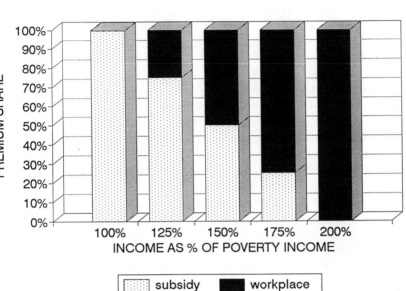

Bibliography

Brown, E.R. 1989. "Access to Health Insurance in the United States," *Medical Care Review* 46(4): 349-385.

Friedman, G. 1989. "New York Effort to Reach Uninsured Falls Short," *Managed Healthcare* 1(3): 10.

Gabel, J., C. Jajich-Toth, G. DeLissovoy, T. Rice, and H. Cohen. 1989. "The Changing World of Group Health Insurance," *Health Affairs* 7(2): 48-65.

Health Management Associates. 1989. *Controlling the Costs of Health Insurance for Small Businesses in Michigan.* Detroit: Independent Business Research Office of Michigan.

Hogan, A.J. 1989. *Report on Small Employee Health Insurance Survey,* presented to the Governor's Task Force on Access to Care. September.

Kramon, G. 1989. "Small Business is Overwhelmed by Health Costs," *New York Times* (October 1).

Moyer, M.E. 1989. "A Revised Look at the Number of Uninsured Americans," *Health Affairs* (Summer).

Perry, L. 1989. "Spending on Primary Care at the Local Level Staves Off Bigger Indigent-Care Costs Later On," *Modern Healthcare* 19(30): 56-62.

Short, P.F., A. Monheit, and K. Beauregard. 1988. *Uninsured Americans: A 1987 Profile.* Rockville, MD: National Center for Health Services Research.

Smith, V.K. 1989. "Health Care Access Project Explores One Solution for the Uninsured," *Michigan Medicine* (April).

Swartz, K. 1989. *The Medically Uninsured: Special Focus on Workers.* Washington, DC: The Urban Institute Press.

Thorpe, K.E., J.E. Siegel, and T. Dailey. 1989. "Including the Poor: The Fiscal Impacts of Medicaid Expansion, *JAMA* 261(7): 1003-1007.

5.3
Medicaid Buy-In Programs for Uninsured Children and Nonworking Adults

Andrew J. Hogan
Stephen A. Woodbury
Michigan State University

Program for Uninsured Children

Characteristics of Uninsured Children

Children under age 19 without health insurance coverage comprise roughly 30 percent of the uninsured population (Short, Monheit, and Beauregard 1988). At least two-thirds of these children in Michigan live in families at less than 200 percent of poverty income and about half of these children live in households where no one has insurance coverage. Another quarter live in families where only the head has coverage. While noninfant children are fairly inexpensive to insure, their low family income levels make it unlikely that universal coverage can be achieved without substantial subsidies. Unfortunately, the existence of a Children's Medicaid Buy-In is likely to induce many small businesses now offering coverage for dependent children to drop that coverage. A few children have nongroup coverage, which their parents would almost certainly drop for the cheaper Buy-In-coverage. Even when a childrens' program is restricted to families where the parents are unemployed or employed in firms eligible for the small business insurance pool, the number of potentially eligible children could expand beyond those currently uninsured.

Rationale for Medicaid Buy-In

Many small businesses that offer health benefits provide at least the option for dependent coverage (SBA 1987; Hogan 1989). As noted above, however, a large percentage of Michigan children are uninsured. Given the likely low participation rate in any small business health insurance pool (Perry 1989), it may be desirable to promote insurance coverage for all children by offering a special Medicaid Buy-In program, if their parents are unemployed, employed in a small business (<25 FTE), or not in the labor force.

Benefit Options

A modest benefit package with some copays and deductibles should cost about $50 per month (1988 dollars).[1] If infants (< 1 year) are excluded from the program, the monthly premium could be cut in half (Blue Cross-Blue Shield Association 1989a, 1989b).

Premium cost-sharing could be based on the family's ability to pay:[2]

$$\text{Premium share} = \frac{\text{Adjusted family income}^2}{\text{Poverty rate income}} - 1. \tag{1}$$

Families above 200 percent of poverty would pay the full premium, while those below 100 percent of poverty would pay no premium (see Figure 1). Substantial subsidies may be necessary to finance the program, since two-thirds of these children are from families with incomes below 200 percent of poverty.

The Unemployed Uninsured Adults Medicaid Buy-In Program

Characteristics of Uninsured Unemployed Adults

This group comprises about 10 percent of the uninsured. Fifty-three percent of this population live in families with less than 200 percent of poverty income. In households with at least on unemployed adult worker, approximately 70 percent of the adults and 95 percent of the children are uninsured.

Figure 1
Premium Shares: Medicaid Buy-In Program
(Nonworking Adults and Children's Pool)

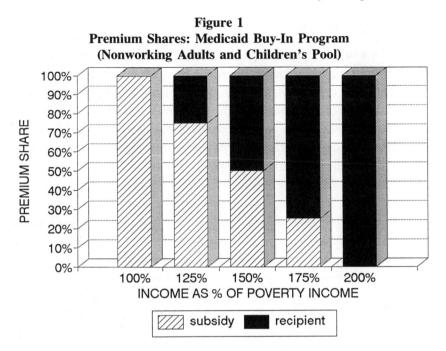

Rationale

It seems unlikely that subsidizing employees to purchase COBRA continuation coverage can be less expensive than the Medicaid Buy-In, since Medicaid payments are so modest. Further, this would be of assistance only to those persons who actually had coverage in their previous employment.

For the unemployed uninsured to buy into the Medicaid program, two options are examined: a subsidized and an unsubsidized program. Eligibility would be determined by the state unemployment insurance agency. Individuals applying for health insurance coverage would need to be actively looking for work, but they need not be receiving unemployment insurance benefits. The health benefit would act as an incentive to continue the job search. However, if large numbers of employers fail to offer health benefits, the unemployed job searcher is likely to remain unemployed for a longer period, and this may increase the cost of unemployment insurance. This will also act as an incentive for employers to offer insurance, at least during times of relative labor shortage.

Benefit Options

The costs of this program vary according to the type of coverage offered. If coverage is provided only to the job searcher, then costs would range from $60 to $100 per individual per month. A more difficult issue is the coverage of spouses and children of the unemployed uninsured. If health insurance coverage is not widely adopted by small businesses, uninsured employed spouses and uninsured children may try to receive coverage via their unemployed spouse/parent. This would create an even greater barrier to accepting a position without health benefits, prolonging unemployment and raising unemployment insurance costs.

Since not all unemployed persons are poor (about 47 percent live in families with incomes above 200 percent of poverty), we suggest for the subsidized option a cost-sharing arrangement in which the uninsured unemployed beneficiary pays a share of the total premium as specified in equation (1). Persons from families at or above 200 percent of poverty would pay the entire premium and persons from families at or below 100 percent of poverty would pay no premium. The majority of unemployed persons will need to have their premiums subsidized, unless the nonpoor unemployed uninsured are charged an actuarially unfair premium sufficient to subsidize the poor (as was attempted with the ill-fated Medicare catastrophic coverage).

Uninsured Not-In-the-Labor-Force (NILF) Adults

Characteristics of Nonworking Adults

Roughly 20 percent of uninsured persons are neither employed nor looking for work. This is, in general, a poor population, with more than 70 percent of the uninsured living in families below 200 percent of poverty.

Rationale for Medicaid Buy-In

A Medicaid Buy-In could be made available for persons not in the labor force. The lack of affordable child care causes many employable women with young children to withdraw from the labor force. If employment-based health insurance or insurance for the unemployed uninsured were not to cover adult dependents, then a significant population group could be left without the opportunity for coverage (as much as 10 percent of the uninsured population). Other unemployed individuals with specific medical problems that make it difficult for them to obtain health insurance elsewhere also may represent a sizable uninsured population. Miscellaneous other individuals, such as the disabled who are not covered by Medicaid or Medicare, may also need health insurance coverage. We suggest a special program for a Medicaid Buy-In for individuals who cannot reasonably be expected to obtain employment-based coverage.

Benefit Options

Again, for the subsidized program, the premium share for individuals is determined by the family income level (see equation 1). The Medicaid Buy-In for normal health risk would cost between $60 and $100 per month. Since 73 percent of this population lives in families with incomes below 200 percent of poverty, substantial subsidies will be necessary to achieve reasonable participation rates. Again, high rates of premium subsidization in combination with low participation rates of emplooyers in a small employer health insurance pool may act as a significant employment disincentive. Selection of a benefit package under the voluntary approach is, by necessity, market driven. The package must be acceptable to those who buy it, but it must not be so rich that it creates more health care cost inflation by causing the coverage offered by firms currently providing benefits to expand, nor should the package be so rich that the unemployed have a disincentive to seek employment. Thus, the package selected should be slightly below that typically offered by small employers.

Administrative Issues

A major difficulty with the voluntary Medicaid Buy-In options presented here is that the beneficiary premium share may need to be paid in after-tax dollars. For an employed population, firms could be asked to create flexible spending accounts into which employees can deposit pre-tax dollars, which then might be used to purchase coverage from the Medicaid Buy-In program. A similar arrangement might be possible for persons receiving unemployment insurance. However, unemployed uninsured who have exhausted their unemployment benefits and those not in the labor force may have to make their premium contributions in after-tax dollars. Deductibility of health care expenses for federal income tax has been limited by recent tax law changes and is available only to itemizers. Other things being equal, to achieve some level of coverage in the currently uninsured population, more state subsidies will be required to compensate for the after-tax cost of the coverage to the nonpoor.

NOTES

1. This premium estimate assumes that catastrophically ill infants would continue to "spend down" to Medicaid eligibility.

2. Adjusted for the value of the premium contribution and the expected deductibles and copayments:

$$\text{Premium share} = \frac{(\text{Family income} - \text{premium} - \text{expected copays and deductibles})}{\text{Poverty income} + \text{premium}} .$$

References

Blue Cross-Blue Shield Association. 1989a. "Syracuse Plans Begin Enrolling Children in Caring Program," *Consumer Exchange* (August).

_____. 1989b. "Insurance Program Created for Needy Ohio Children," *Consumer Exchange* (September).

Danzon, P.M. 1989. "Mandated Employment-Based Health Insurance: Incidence and Efficiency Effects," unpublished manuscript.

Hogan, A.J. 1989. *Small Employer Health Insurance Survey: A Report to the Governor's Task Force on Access to Health Care* (October).

Perry, L. 1989. "Spending on Primary Care at Local Level Staves Off Bigger Indigent Care Costs Later On," *Modern Healthcare* 19(30): 56-62, July 28.

Short, P.F., A. Monheit, and K. Beauregard. 1988. *Uninsured Americans: A 1987 Profile,* Rockville, MD: National Center for Health Services Research.

Small Business Administration (SBA). 1987. "Health Care Coverage and Costs in Small and Large Business," *The State of Small Business, 1987,* Washington, DC.

5.4
High-Risk Pools

Dianne Miller Wolman
Wayne State University

High-risk pools are created by states to expand the availability of private health insurance for individuals who have serious medical conditions and have difficulty purchasing insurance. Such pools are relatively attractive politically as a mechanism for reducing the size of the uninsured population in a state and do, in fact, permit some medically (not economically) needy individuals to purchase health insurance.

There is a sizable and growing population of individuals with medical conditions or past medical experiences that indicate the potential for high medical bills in the future. Private insurance companies consider these people "bad risks" and may substantially increase their premium, exclude treatment for the pre-existing condition, or refuse to sell them insurance (Griss 1988, p. 43). Such actions make it impractical or impossible for some people to buy coverage, particularly if they are not part of a group plan. Estimates of the size of this population vary, but they are often in the vicinity of 1 percent of the total population or 1 percent of the under 65 population (Bovbjerg and Koller 1986, p. 111; Intergovernmental Health Policy Project 1988, p. 13). The Health Insurance Survey of Michigan found that 1.5 percent of the state's total population had no insurance, ranked their health status as fair or poor, and/or felt they had a disabling condition (Bashshur, Webb, and Homan 1989). There is agreement that, regardless of the precise size of this population today, it is growing and will continue to for the foreseeable future.

The numbers of the difficult-to-insure are growing for several reasons. First, early detection and medical treatments are increasing the survival rates for many diseases. Second, screening programs are detecting

This work was performed under the sponsorship of the Board of Governors of Wayne State University and the College of Urban, Labor and Metropolitan Affairs.

diseases at earlier stages, before symptoms become evident (U.S. Congress 1988a,b). Third, competitive pressures on insurers to hold down premiums lead them to reduce risks by taking action when possible against those with specific, known medical conditions. And, fourth, employers are under pressure to minimize their costs and are tempted to take corresponding actions against the same individuals. Future trends in medical technology and health care cost inflation point toward an expanding population of the medically uninsurable. High-risk pools appear to be an obvious answer to this problem.

What Is a High-Risk Pool and How Does It Work?

Organization

The general structure of high-risk pools is similar from state to state, although there is some variation in the details. The pool is created by state legislation, which forms an association of all health insurance companies doing business in the state and establishes an independent governing board. Some states also require health maintenance organizations (HMOs) to participate. Self-insured plans are not included because of their exemption from state regulation under the Employee Retirement Income Security Act of 1974 (ERISA). The pool is governed by a board including representatives of the insurance industry, state government officials, and consumers. It is responsible for setting the package of benefits, recommending premium rates, and contracting with a private insurance company to administer the program on a daily basis as the lead carrier. Insurance agents receive a fee fixed by the pool for enrolling new members. It is less than a commission would be and provides some savings on administrative costs. The state insurance department provides oversight for the program.

Benefit Package

The enabling legislation generally requires the pool to offer insurance coverage of a full and traditional range of major medical services similar to that offered in large group plans. The benefits are not designed specifically to include all the providers and treatments often needed by individuals with chronic and/or handicapping conditions, just those standard for acute medical care. Where there are service limits, they tend to be relatively high and provider reimbursement is reasonable. There is a maximum limit on total dollar lifetime benefits and also annual limits on out-of-pocket spending (stop/loss). Copayments are usually at 20 percent, and there are deductibles with amounts that vary from state to state. Some pools offer different deductible levels, depending on which option/premium level the enrollee chooses (see Table 1). Some states include in their benefit package some cost-containment mechanisms, such as utilization controls.

Premium

The state enabling legislation imposes a limit on the premiums that can be charged. The maximum is a percentage (generally 150 percent) of the average premium rates for standard health risks with comparable coverage (see Table 2). The premiums are rated for age and sex. While the pools start with premiums below the maximum, they rapidly increase to the limit as the costs become evident.

Financing

Most pools operate at a loss because the utilization and health care costs of high-risk individuals are significantly greater than 150 percent of the average, but their premiums are capped. The losses most often are paid by the member insurance companies, based on their market share in the state. In a few states, the companies must treat this assessment as part of the costs of doing business in the state. Elsewhere, the companies are permitted a credit against their state tax bills for the full assessment (see Table 2).

Eligibility

The pools are designed primarily for the medically "uninsurable" and require evidence from the applicant of that status. They reject the insurance concept of spreading the risk broadly across a heterogeneous population and anticipate the inevitable adverse selection. Even states

Table 1
State High-Risk Pools: Eligibility and Benefit Structure

State	Eligibility	Benefit package for individual		
		Deductibles ($)	Out-of-pocket annual limit ($)	Lifetime maximum ($)
Connecticut	All residents ineligible for Medicare	400-1,500	2,000	1,000,000
Florida	Resident ineligible for Medicaid, plus Rejected by 2 insurers, Received notice of benefit reduction, or Premium increase exceeded pool rate	1,000-2,000	2,500-3,500	500,000
Illinois	Residents ineligible for Medicaid, plus Rejected by 1 insurer, Premium increase exceeded pool rate, or Certain medical conditions covered automatically Also, groups of 10 or less if 1 or more meets above criteria	250-1,500	1,500	500,000
Indiana	Residents ineligible for Medicare, plus Rejected by 2 insurers, Received notice of benefit reduction, Premium increase exceeded pool rate, or Certain medical conditions covered automatically	200-1,000	1,000-2,000	none 50,000 limit on mental and nervous disorders
Iowa	Residents ineligible for Medicaid, plus Rejected by 1 insurer, Premium exceeded pool rate, or Certain medical conditions covered automatically	500-1,000	1,500-2,000	250,000
Maine	Residents ineligible for Medicare or Medicaid, plus Premium exceeded pool rate	500-1,000	5,000	250,000

State	Eligibility criteria			
Minnesota	Rejected by 1 insurer, Restrictive rider limits coverage, Premium exceeded pool rate, or Certain medical conditions covered automatically	500–1,000	3,000	500,000
Montana	Rejected by 2 insurers, or Restrictive rider limits coverage	500–1,000	5,000	250,000
Nebraska	Residents ineligible for Medicare or Medicaid, plus Rejected by 1 insurer, Restrictive rider limits coverage, or Premium exceeded pool rate	250–1,000 (10% co-insurance)	5,000	500,000
New Mexico	Residents ineligible for Medicare or Medicaid, plus Rejected by 1 insurer, Restrictive rider limits coverage, or Premium exceeded pool rate	500–1,000	1,500–2,000	none
N. Dakota	Rejected by 1 insurer, or Restrictive rider limits coverage	150–1,000	3,000	250,000
Tennessee	Residents ineligible for Medicaid, plus Rejected by 1 insurer	500–2,000	1,500–2,500	500,000
Washington	Residents ineligible for Medicaid, plus Rejected by 1 insurer, or Restrictive rider limits coverage	500–1,000	1,500–2,500	500,000
Wisconsin	Residents ineligible for Medicaid, plus Rejected by 1 insurer, or Received notice of benefit reduction, or Premium exceeded pool rate	1,000 (deductible subsidized for low-income individuals)	500–2,000	500,000

SOURCES: Communicating for Agriculture, Inc. 1988; Intergovernmental Health Policy Project 1988, p. 5; and U.S. General Accounting Office 1988, pp. 11-14.

Table 2
State High-Risk Pools: Financial Features, 1989

State, date operational	Enrollment	Premium cap (percent)*	Premiums collected ($)	Claims paid ($)	Pool funding mechanism
Connecticut 1976	2,127	125-150	3,460,000	6,565,000	-insurers assessed; tax credit
Florida 1983	4,849	150-200	4,618,650	8,582,000	-insurers assessed; tax credit removed 1989 -limit on assessments: ≤1% of health insurance premiums written in state
Illinois 1989	2,560	135	NA	NA	-legislative appropriation of general revenues
Indiana 1982	2,610	150	5,607,908	9,640,519	-insurers assessed; tax credit
Iowa 1987	1,495	150	1,197,800	1,250,000	-insurers assessed; tax credit
Maine 1988	109 (300 enrollees maximum set by legislature)	125	15,178	0	-new tax of up to .0015% on hospital gross patient services revenue
Minnesota 1976	14,386	125	14,197,219	27,098,596	-insurers and HMOs assessed; no tax credit since 1987

Montana 1987	109	150-400	97,026	65,374	-insurers assessed; tax credit
Nebraska 1986	1,750	135-165	6,005	185,000	-insurers assessed; tax credit
New Mexico 1988	698	150	233,053	127,399	-insurers assessed; no tax credit until member's assessment ≥$75,000, then 30% credit allowed for excess amount over $75,000
N. Dakota 1982	1,551	135	1,197,903	3,340,441	-insurers assessed; tax credit
Tennessee 1987	3,933	135-150	2,794,650	2,807,000	-insurers assessed; tax credit -state cap of $3 million/yr. on state funds to pay pool costs
Washington 1988	1,153	150	385,100	18,680	-insurers assessed; tax credit
Wisconsin 1981	4,497	150 (premium subsidy for low-income individuals)	4,056,671	5,518,189	-insurers assessed; no tax credit -$200,000 tax relief from general revenues as of 1/1/88

SOURCES: Burda 1989, p. 54; Communicating for Agriculture, Inc. 1988; Intergovernmental Health Policy Project 1988; Marvin 1990; and Trippler 1990.
*These percentages represent the limit on pool premiums relative to the average premium charged in the state for comparable policies for standard health risks.

that permit normal-risk applicants to enroll expect primarily high-risk individuals. Adverse selection tends to have a snowball effect and eventually drives out normal-risk individuals who can find lower premiums elsewhere.

What Has Been the Impact of High-Risk Pools?

Historical Growth

The first high-risk pools were created in Connecticut and Minnesota in 1976, and since then 17 more states have passed enabling legislation. Of those 19, 5 are not yet operational—California, Georgia, Oregon, South Carolina and Texas. Many states are currently considering such legislation (Marvin 1990). The concept is popular politically because the high-risk pool appears to serve a needy and deserving population, is operated through the private sector, and provides an indirect and seemingly limited role for the state government. However, while there may be no public discussion of a sizable appropriation to fund the pool's deficit, legislators are becoming more aware of the financing limitations of the traditional pool concept and the implications of the tax credit.

Costs and Losses

As pool enrollments grow, so do their losses. This may not be a serious problem during the first years of a program, in part because of pre-existing conditions clauses and the normal time lag of medical bills. Also, the total deficit starts out relatively small because there are few enrollees. However, the average enrollee generates greater costs than the premium he or she pays—even in Connecticut, where more normal risks are included in the pool. The 14 pools operating in 1988 showed a total of more than $65 million in claims paid compared to $39 million in premiums collected (Burda 1989, p. 54). (See Table 2.) Administrative costs of 12 to 15 percent of total pool spending increase the deficits even more (Bovbjerg and Koller 1986, p. 118).

The claims costs per enrollee vary widely, depending in part upon the maturity of the program and the medical cost index in each geographic area. Minnesota found that 1 percent of its enrollment generated 30 percent of its claims costs. Such data are unavailable for other states. Since Minnesota has less adverse selection than some states because of its relatively low premiums, it may have a relatively large group that generates few claims. Nonetheless, it is likely in all pools that a small portion of enrollees generate a disproportionately large share of the costs (Trippler 1990).

Cost Burden

It is not entirely obvious who bears the costs of the high-risk pools. The premium, which is itself only part of total costs, is normally paid by the enrollee (except in Wisconsin and Maine, where the state provides a direct subsidy of premiums for low-income enrollees). However, some enrollees have their premium paid by their employers. In some states, there are indications that 15 to 20 percent of the pool's enrollees may have such an arrangement. This means that employers and perhaps their group insurers are taking advantage of the existence of a high-risk pool to off-load their high-risk employees and to keep their group plan costs at a more reasonable level. The employer and other employees benefit because the premiums will be lower without high-cost employee members. Also, high-risk workers seeking employment do not have to fear discrimination in hiring based on employers' fears about high group medical costs.

On the other hand, the state is usually picking up the deficits from those high-risk employees who previously had been covered privately. Certainly, many pool boards are very concerned about this phenomenon (Marvin 1990).

Since the premium covers substantially less than the full program costs, who pays the deficit? In the states that permit the insurance companies to offset their assessment as a tax credit, the result is a dollar-for-dollar reduction of general revenues. It represents a tax expenditure and its effect is the same as a direct appropriation. Hence, the taxpayers in the state bear that burden. Tennessee's recently passed legislation places a limit of $3 million on annual pool costs to the state. In states such as Minnesota, which eliminated the tax credit for pool deficits, the insurers bear the deficits as a cost of doing business. Thus, the insurance companies' owners and/or customers (employers, employees and private, nongroup enrollees) pay the extra costs. Members of self-insured plans are unaffected. Those plans are growing in popularity, to some extent because of their competitive advantage. Illinois and Wisconsin recently passed legislation to fund all or part of the deficit through an appropriation of general revenues, and thus the burden is spread broadly across all taxpayers. Maine funds its deficit by a new tax on hospital gross patient services revenue, so the cost is shifted to hospital users who pay their own bills and to third parties and their enrollees.

Enrollment Growth

Although there have been fluctuations in enrollment within pools, in total, there has been steady, moderate growth over the years. The latest enrollment figures show almost 42,000 individuals covered nationally (Burda 1989, p. 54). (See Table 2.) That is a small fraction of the medically uninsurable population, an estimated two to three million in the U.S. It is also much less than those who could afford to join (Fraser 1988, p. 202). Clearly, annual premiums of several thousand dollars are a barrier to all but those with middle- to upper-level incomes. And only 30 to 40 percent of the uninsured have incomes above $20,000. Nevertheless, the participation of those with sufficient income is also low, perhaps because the marketing of the pools has not been very effective.

While the total enrollment of 42,000 seems low, it underestimates the total number of individuals served, since it is reflective of only one point in time. More individuals are served during the year as many move in and out of the program. For example, a high-risk individual would drop out if he or she became eligible for group coverage from a new job. The exact turnover rate in various pools is unknown, since most pools collect very little administrative data.

Cost-Containment

By definition, the high-risk pools suffer from adverse selection and have a relatively large share of heavy users of health services. Given their high volume and cost of services, cost-containment mechanisms are crucial to high-risk pools. Unfortunately, only half the pools have used cost controls as a standard part of their administrative practices (U.S. General Accounting Office 1988). They have adopted a few selected cost-containment measures, such as preadmission certification for hospital care and second surgical opinion programs. However, much remains to be done in all the pools to initiate efforts to ensure effectively and efficiently run programs.

What Are Policy Issues to Consider Before Initiating a Pool?

Is There an Insurer of Last Resort in the State?

Eleven states and the District of Columbia require Blue Cross-Blue Shield plans to offer open enrollment for individual (nongroup) coverage. The plans are not permitted to discriminate according to health status. If the premiums charged for this coverage are state-regulated as closely as would be a pool's premiums, there would be little need for a separate high-risk pool. If the state does not have an open enrollment regulation, it might be worth examining the operation of this regulation in other states to determine whether it might be feasible and preferable to a high-risk pool. It is important to consider how and by whom the excessive costs of high-risk members would be covered in such an arrangement. Note that the existence of an open enrollment requirement does not provide a total solution to the medically uninsurable problem. It has the same limitation as does the pool—expensive premiums.

How Does the State Regulate Insurance Underwriting Currently?

The medically uninsurable population is defined, to some extent, by the insurance industry, which is regulated by the state. The existence and nature of restrictions placed on underwriting practices, methods for defining group plans, and so forth, can affect both the population left without coverage and the reaction of employers to the creation of a high-risk pool. For example, can employers and/or insurers define the members of a group plan based on the health status of individuals? Are insurers limited in the medical screening they can do? Can pre-existing conditions be excluded from coverage when an employer switches plans?

Who Would Pay the Pool Losses and How Visible Should the Mechanism Be?

Ultimately this will be a political issue, but it is also useful to analyze it explicitly during the development of the proposal. It must be recognized from the start that losses are inevitable and will grow as the pool more successfully serves its target population.

How Can the State Promote Equitable Treatment of Both Private Insurance Plans and Self-Insured Groups?

The choice of financing mechanisms will affect the balance. Until federal legislation is passed to change the ERISA exemption, indirect methods and taxes may be necessary if the state wants to tap a broader funding source than just the private insurance plans.

What Should Be the State's Position Concerning the Shift of High-Risk Individuals from Employer Plans to the High-Risk Pool?

If the state is aware of the advantages and disadvantages of such shifting from the private sector to the public, it could design pool details, such as regulatory controls, monitoring mechanisms, or employer taxes to create an equitable impact. Basically, is it preferable for the costs of employed high-risk individuals to be covered privately through employer groups or publicly through the pool's premium and deficit? What are the state's broader goals concerning private employer coverage?

What Cost-Containment Mechanisms Could Help Limit the Pool's Losses?

The state could look to efficiently run private and Blue Cross-Blue Shield insurance plans in its area, as well as to the current evaluation literature to see what mechanisms work and might be suitable to its population, medical providers, and so forth. Some administrative procedures and controls might be built into the benefit package and administrative program during development, while others require a critical mass of enrollees in order to be practical.

Are the Pool Costs (Losses) Worth the Benefits in Terms of State Health Priorities and Population Needs?

Is a high-risk pool just a politically attractive, "doable" program compared to other proposals for the uninsured, or is it really serving high-priority needs? Are the higher-priority programs not feasible at the moment and does the pool appear worthwhile even if of limited impact on the numbers of uninsured? Could the pool's deficit dollars be better spent on Medicaid expansion or a public health service program for poor children? Would those dollars be available for these possibly higher-priority populations?

Could the High-Risk Pool Be Adapted to Serve Other Priority Needs?

What kind of premium subsidies would be necessary to serve the medically uninsurable of low-to-moderate income who are not covered by Medicaid? Where would the money come from? Could the premiums be reduced by opening the pool to the uninsured of normal risk, and what changes would be necessary to attract them?

Conclusions

High-risk pools have been in operation since the late 1970s. None have failed. All have grown and are successfully making private health insurance available to those who can pay the premium. However, their costs to the public are not insignificant, though they are frequently not obvious. Also, while the program serves a politically attractive population, it may not be meeting a high-priority policy need. The political and administrative costs as well as financial costs and time necessary to create and operate a high-risk pool should be weighed against the expected benefits from such a program. If it is a useful program for the state, care should be taken in the policy development process to incorporate effective cost controls, premium subsidies if necessary to serve priority populations, and an equitable financing mechanism.

References

Bashshur, Rashid, Cater Webb, and Rick Homan. 1989. ''Health Insurance Survey of Michigan on Access to Health Care.'' School of Public Health, University of Michigan, Ann Arbor. Photocopy.

Bovbjerg, Randall R. and Christopher F. Koller. 1986. ''State Health Insurance Pools: Current Performance, Future Prospects.'' *Inquiry* 23 (Summer): 111-121.

Burda, David. 1989. ''Risk Pools Are Filling Coverage Needs of People Who Can Afford Health Insurance But Can't Get It.'' *Modern Healthcare* (July 28): 45-56.

Communicating for Agriculture, Inc. 1988. *Comprehensive Health Insurance for High-Risk Individuals*. Minneapolis: CA Support Services Office.

Fraser, Irene. 1988. *Promoting Health Insurance in the Workplace: State and Local Initiatives to Increase Private Coverage*. Chicago: American Hospital Association.

Griss, Bob. 1988. *Access to Health Care*. Washington, DC: World Institute on Disability, September.

Intergovernmental Health Policy Project. 1988. ''The Risk Pool Strategy: Comprehensive Health Insurance Associations.'' *Focus On...* 20 (February).

Marvin, George. 1990. Telephone conversation with author, 24 January.

Trippler, Aaron. 1990. Telephone conversation with author, 31 January.

U.S. Congress, Office of Technology Assessment. 1988a. *AIDS and Health Insurance*. Washington, DC: Government Printing Office, February.

_____. 1988b. *Medical Testing and Health Insurance, Summary*. Washington, DC: Government Printing Office, August.

U.S. General Accounting Office. 1988. *Health Insurance—Risk Pools for the Medically Uninsurable*. Briefing Report to the Committee on Labor and Human Resources, U.S. Senate. Washington, DC: Government Printing Office, April.

5.5
Uncompensated Care
What States Are Doing
John M. Herrick
Joseph Papsidero
Michigan State University

Since the early 1980s, the problem of providing access to health care for those who cannot afford it has received considerable attention. Nonuniform Medicaid eligibility policies across states have resulted in less than 40 percent of those below the federal poverty line being eligible for Medicaid (Bautista 1986; Burwell and Rymer 1987; Jones 1989). A population estimated to number as many as 37 million is without health insurance (Bashshur and Webb, chapter 2 in this volume). The absence of inclusive federal policies and programs to provide health care access for at-risk populations has left the states with the responsibility of addressing the problems of access to care for those who cannot pay.

Hospitals have traditionally provided uncompensated care, defined as charity care and bad debt losses, and shifted the costs of such care to patients who had private insurance or Medicare (Saywell et al. 1989; Hadley and Feder 1985). It has been estimated that because of cost-shifting, private payers paid an average of 10.6 percent more for hospital-based care in 1982 (Hadley and Feder 1985; King 1989). Today, cost-shifting has become more difficult since payers have instituted various cost-containment procedures. But uncompensated care has continued to be provided by many hospitals, and its costs have escalated.

Measuring the volume of uncompensated care is problematic because of ambiguities in defining what is uncompensated and difficulties in determining the actual costs of care. Estimates of dollar amounts of uncompensated care have often not distinguished between provider *charges* for care and the actual *costs* of that care, resulting in nonuniform estimates. Nonetheless, one estimate of the cost of care for which hospitals were not compensated directly and which was not covered by government appropriations indicates that it climbed from $2.8 billion to $7.2 billion between 1980 and 1987 (King 1989). In 1988, the American Hospital Association (1990) estimated that 6,438 nonprofit and state and local government hospitals provided a total of $14.6 billion of uncompensated care.

Hospitals, in a competitive environment, adopt cost-containment strategies which may include limiting or eliminating uncompensated care to those without financial access. The American Hospital Association found in 1981 and 1982 that nearly 15 percent of hospitals surveyed limited the amount of charity care they provided. That included 26 percent of public hospitals that were members of the Council of Teaching Hospitals (Glenn 1985; Jones 1989). Financially stressed hospitals, in order to control costs, may engage in "patient dumping," leaving public hospitals and those with historic commitments to serve the poor with the challenge of trying to provide quality care to those who are unable to fully pay for services received. The net result is increased risk for those who are uninsured or underinsured.

State Responses

State responses to the issue of uncompensated care vary. The following examples demonstrate some of the differences in state initiatives.

Florida

Florida attempted to deal with uncompensated care in its Health Care Access Act of 1984 (HCAA). The Act established a medically indigent pool funded by an assessment on hospital net operating revenue and a state contribution. This pool would provide the nonfederal match for expanding Medicaid. Hospitals were not targeted directly for uncompensated care reimbursement, since it was felt that in reporting amounts of uncompensated care they could include bad debt, charity care, contractual allowances, professional "courtesy" care and third-party discounts, making estimates of revenues lost because of care for the uninsured or underinsured unreliable. The unreliability of such data contributed to the political decision to focus on consumers by expanding Medicaid and medically needy programs, and by committing funds to primary health care programs (Jones 1989; Lewin 1985). Hospitals that chose to serve patients covered under these expanded programs could attempt to recoup revenues lost through the assessment. Evaluations of the Health Care Access Act reveal it did not solve the problem of provision of uncompensated care. Certain hospitals admitted more Medicaid patients but continued their practices of denying access to those who were uninsured (Jones 1989).

In 1987, Florida passed the Indigent Care Bill to provide financial support to hospitals providing disproportionate amounts of care to the poor. It attempted to establish an equitable method for distributing the burden of indigent care among providers. It also provided higher rates of reimbursement to physicians for certain procedures, such as obstetrical services, in an attempt to improve access to care for the poor using some of the funds collected by the assessment on hospital net revenues. Florida has seen an increase in the demand for uncompensated care, resulting in heavier burdens for financing and delivering uncompensated care for a decreasing number of providers as alternative medical care delivery modalities increase. Jones (1989) suggests the need for better long-term public and private insurance solutions to the uncompensated care problem, as well as a physician "tax" raised by a surcharge on licensing fees as a means of providing funds to support indigent care programs.

Florida's efforts are attempts to equitably distribute financing of indigent care without the regulatory approach of an all-payer system. It employs hospital assessments, Medicaid expansions, use of medically needy and medically indigent programs, and an experimental effort to make health insurance accessible to small employers (Jones 1989).

In contrast to Florida's mixed-approach, other states have addressed uncompensated care through "all-payer" and other approaches. A brief overview of actions taken by these states to deal with uncompensated care follows. A basic assumption of all-payer systems is that the state assumes control of hospital costs by instituting rate-setting, and that all purchasers of care at a particular hospital are to pay the same rates.

Maryland

Since the early 1970s, hospital reimbursement rates have been regulated in Maryland. In 1977, the state requested and was granted all-payer waiver status by the federal government. This was part of a state strategy to improve access to health care while at the same time attempting to control health care costs. The Maryland Health Services Cost Review Commission was charged with establishing prospective rates for specific services and procedures. Hospitals were to be reimbursed for provision of uncompensated care after review of their requests. If the request was approved, the costs of uncompensated care became part of the rates that all payers were required to pay for services at that hospital. This process assures that all payers for hospital services share the reasonable costs of uncompensated care (Salkever, Steinwachs and Rupp 1986). In effect, this approach spread the costs of uncompensated care among all payers, thereby increasing its political feasibility. Davidson (1985) admits Maryland's approach has its critics, but argues that it does seem to provide access to health care for Maryland's residents, including those whose care had previously been uncompensated. He found that in 1983, nearly all Maryland inner-city hospitals providing relatively large amounts of uncompensated care were profit making. Medicaid patients may also have gained access to more providers than previously, thereby offering greater freedom of choise. Thus, Maryland's all-payer system, despite problems, may have gone far towards finding a workable method for dealing with the problem of uncompensated care for the poor and uninsured.

New Jersey

New Jersey's all-payer rate-setting system began in the 1980s. In order to provide access to health care for those without insurance, the state allowed hospitals to include charity care and bad debt losses as reimbursable costs, thereby providing incentives for hospitals to treat the uninsured. Rosko (1990) found that New Jersey's all-payer system has increased access to inpatient and outpatient hospital care to the uninsured. It has also provided needed financial support to inner-city and teaching hospitals, which have historically provided considerable amounts of uncompensated care (Halpern 1985). There are many questions regarding the financial impact of all-payer systems on hospitals that can be addressed but that are beyond the scope of this brief overview.[1]

New Jersey's hospitals share in the total cost of uncompensated care. Insurance premiums, paid by employees and private-pay patients, include payment for uncompensated care. In 1988, it was estimated that New Jersey's uncompensated care costs were nearly $400 million. Under New Jersey's all-payer system, most third-party payers cover the costs of uncompensated care in the rates they pay for hospital care. In effect, a surcharge is added to hospital bills. Excess revenue goes to the state's Uncompensated Care Trust Fund, administered by the New Jersey Department of Health, which then pays hospitals that provide above average amounts of uncompensated care. Medicaid also assists in funding uncompensated care, since federal law requires state Medicaid agencies to provide additional amounts to hospitals with relatively large amounts of uncompensated care (New Jersey 1989; Rosko 1989).

New Jersey has found that total uncompensated care expenses have risen recently (Rosko 1990). It has been suggested that this may be because of hospitals opting not to aggressively collect on bad debts, since they can seek reimbursement from the uncompensated care fund. If New Jersey's approach to dealing with uncompensated care is to continue, it must maintain political viability, which could be weakened if uncompensated care costs became viewed as unmanageable. New Jersey's system has improved access to hospital care, but it does not guarantee that all uninsured persons will in fact receive such care. Individuals may still be unable or unwilling to attempt to gain access to hospitals because they may seem inaccessible and forbidding. The acceptability of medical services to potential patients is another important factor in determining access to services.

Massachusetts

Massachusetts also developed an all-payer system which attempted to reimburse hospitals for uncompensated care in the early 1980s. When Massachusetts initiated its all-payer program, it hoped that medical costs could be controlled and that hospitals that were at risk financially and that may have been providing large amounts of uncompensated care would benefit by plans to reimburse a portion of the costs of that care. Rosenbloom (1985), in assessing the Massachusetts all-payer system, concluded that its main purpose was to benefit at-risk hospitals, not necessarily to create a program of guaranteed access to health care for the uninsured. Consequently, he cautioned that the system could be used to shield inefficient hospitals, such as those with excess bed capacities.

Many controversial issues arose in Massachusetts in the mid-1980s as the debate over how best to finance uncompensated care intensified. Hospitals providing uncompensated care for the uninsured felt they were competitively disadvantaged, compared to free-standing clinics or surgery centers. In 1985, the Massachusetts Hospital Association argued against continuing the federal waiver which allowed Medicare participation in the all-payer system. Hospitals feared federal limitation on payments, which would increase their financial problems. Eventually, the all-payer approach was discarded. A bad-debt free-care pool was established to reimburse hospitals for uncompensated care. As special interests clamored for or against regulation of health care, the Massachusetts legislature and Governor Dukakis passed the Massachusetts Health Care Security Act in 1988. It intended to provide access to health care for all residents through health insurance. A health insurance trust fund was to be established to provide coverage for the uninsured. The Massachusetts plan will be financed by requiring most employers to pay a surcharge on employees' wages, which will go into a state health insurance trust fund. A new state department will provide health insurance for many uninsured residents. Since 1988, the financial problems of Massachusetts have worsened, leaving uncertain its ability to finance a universal access plan (Goldberger 1990).

New York

New York's approach to the provision of uncompensated care is complex. Like Massachusetts, New Jersey, and Maryland, it utilized an all-payer rate-setting program aimed at controlling hospital costs, financing uncompensated care, and reducing cost-shifting. Eventually, New York developed an insurance-pool approach to promote health care access. Uncompensated care pools, financed through hospital rate-setting, were created to provide access for the uninsured (Berman 1985). Hospitals seeking reimbursement for uncompensated care must demonstrate reasonable efforts to collect bad debts (Meyer 1986). Provider reimbursement for uncompensated care has sometimes proven to be a complex and cumbersome process. Thorpe (1988) analyzed New York's experience and found a "leaky basket effect" in which money earmarked for reimbursement of uncompensated care was used for other purposes. Nevertheless, New York's approach has provided improved access to health care (Rosko 1990).

Summary

Early evaluations of the Maryland and New Jersey all-payer systems suggest they are able to control overall provider costs at least as well as partial-payer systems. Funding mechanisms for uncompensated care reimbursement also promote access to health care for the uninsured. Rosko (1989) found these all-payer systems provide important financial relief to hospitals that provided disproportionate amounts of uncompensated care. Cost-shifting was also reduced. New York's complex system appears to have produced similar results (Thorpe 1987).

All-payer systems are not without potential problems.[2] Service utilization, unless carefully scrutinized, might escalate under such plans, thereby driving overall health care costs upward. All-payer systems should not inadvertently discourage efficient financial management by providers (Wilensky 1986; Meyer 1986). Maryland and New Jersey require hospitals to vigorously attempt to collect on bad debts.

As Feingold (1988) has argued, both quality of care and cost efficiency should be goals of any reimbursement system established to deal with uncompensated care. All-payer systems are attractive, since all insurers or payers would pay identical rates for services offered at specific hospitals. Payment rates can be determined by the state working with providers, consumers and other interested parties. Reimbursement rates can foster payment for the amount of uncompensated care done by a specific hospital.

Among the all-payer systems implemented, there have really been two different stategies used to pay for uncompensated care. One approach builds the costs of such care provided by a particular hospital into the rates that hospital charges and requires all payers using that hospital to pay those rates. This strategy has the apparent disadvantage that hospitals providing a great deal of uncompensated care will need to charge high rates and may have difficulty attracting paying patients in a competitive environment.

The other approach includes a uniform surcharge on rates at all hospitals, with the revenue pooled and redistributed to hospitals providing uncompensated care. It is important to note that, while this strategy has been associated with all-payer systems, it does not, in principle, require such a system. All-payers might pay a uniform surcharge without necessarily paying the same rates for hospital care.

Concluding Remarks

In the absence of a federal program to guarantee access to health care for the uninsured, it is clear that it will be a state and local government responsibility to deal with the problem. Short of establishing a state program of universal coverage, it is also clear that the provision of reimbursement for uncompensated care will be a necessary component of those solutions.

Whereas the foregoing has addressed uncompensated care provided by hospitals, another important aspect is that of uncompensated care provided by physicians. Issues related to uncompensated care by physicians have received relatively little attention in state initiatives. A review of available knowledge about the provision of uncompensated care by physicians showed that there is very little useful data. Available national estimates are limited. However, if these crude estimates are applied at the state level, the contribution of uncompensated care by physicians could be substantial. In contrast to hospitals, which have received some support from insurers to cover the costs of uncompensated care, it appears that such support is not explicitly reflected in payments to physicians.

The lack of useful information may be one of the reasons why uncompensated care by physicians is minimally recognized in state strategies, where the main attention is upon uncompensated care provided by hospitals. Information systems that collect hospital-based data are available, and these sources can be used to derive estimates of the magnitude of uncompensated care. In contrast, there appear to be no information systems for the collection of physician-related data on which to make such estimates.

Our experience in a small preliminary survey indicated that there is great variability in the way physicians report uncompensated care in terms of both "charity care" and "bad debts." Since most physician offices do not appear to have computerized records, the tendency to make rough estimates contributes to the variability and unreliability of such reports. Methods that provide improved information are needed in order to understand uncompensated care provided by physicians.

NOTES

1. See Hsiao and Dunn (1987) for discussion of the impact of New Jersey's all-payer DRG system on hospital costs.

2. Indeed, Massachusetts, New Jersey, and New York have all allowed the Medicare waivers for their all-payer systems to expire.

References

American Hospital Association. 1990. Annual Survey of Hospitals, 1988 estimated file, in *Nonprofit Hospitals: Better Standards Needed for Tax Exemption* (GAO/HRD-90-84). Washington, DC: General Accounting Office.

Bautista, A.S. 1986. "AHA Explored the Cost of Compassion." *Health Law Vigil* 9(11): 7-8.

Berman, Richard A. 1985. "New York." In Sally J. Rogers, et al., *Hospitals and the Uninsured Poor: Measuring and Paying for Uncompensated Care.* New York: United Hospital Fund of New York.

Burwell, B.O. and M.P. Rymer. 1987. "Trends in Medicaid Eligibility: 1975-1985." *Health Affairs* 6(4): 30-45.

Butler, P.A. 1985. "New Initiatives in Financing and Delivering Health Care for the Medically Indigent: Report on a Conference." *Law, Medicare and Health* 13(5): 225-232.

Davidson, Richard J. 1985. "Maryland." In Sally J. Rogers, et al., *Hospitals and the Uninsured Poor: Measuring and Paying for Uncompensated Care.* New York: United Hospital Fund of New York.

Feingold, Eugene. 1988. "What Other States are Doing About Access." *Michigan Hospitals* (June): 9-10, 13, 15.

Glenn, K., ed. 1985. *Medicine and Health/Perspectives.* Washington, DC: McGraw-Hill.

Goldberger, Susan A. 1990. "The Politics of Uninsured Access: The Massachusetts Health Security Act of 1988." *Journal of Health Politics, Policy and Law* 15: 857-885.

Hadley, J. and J. Feder. 1985. "Hospitals Cost Shifting and Care for the Uninsured." *Health Affairs* 4: 67-80.

Halpern, Kevin G. 1985. "New Jersey." In Sally J. Rogers, et al., *Hospitals and the Uninsured Poor: Measuring and Paying for Uncompensated Care.* New York: United Hospital Fund of New York.

Hsaio, William C. and Daniel C. Dunn. 1987. "The Impact of DRG Payment on New Jersey Hospitals." *Inquiry* 24: 212-220.

Jones, Kathleen R. 1989. "The Florida Health Care Access Act: A Blended Regulatory Approach to the Indigent Health Care Problem." *Journal of Health Politics, Policy and Law* 14(2): 261-285.

King, Martha P. 1989. *Medicaid Indigency and Uncompensated Health Care Costs.* Denver: National Conference of State Legislatures.

Lewin, Lawrence S. 1985. "Florida." In Sally J. Rogers, et al., *Hospitals and the Uninsured Poor: Measuring and Paying for Uncompensated Care.* New York: United Hospital Fund of New York.

Meyer, Jack A. 1986. "Financing Uncompensated Care with All-Payer Rate Regulation." In Frank A. Sloan, et al., *Uncompensated Care, Rights and Responsibilities*. Baltimore: Johns Hopkins University Press.

"New Jersey Trust Fund Ensures Access to Hospital Care." 1989. *Public Health Macroview* 2: 7-8.

Rosenbloom, David L. 1985. "Massachusetts." In Sally J. Rogers, et al., *Hospitals and the Uninsured Poor: Measuring and Paying for Uncompensated Care*. New York: United Hospital Fund of New York.

Rosko, Michael D. 1989. "A Comparison of Hospital Performance Under the Partial-Payer Medicare PPS and State All-Payer Rate-Setting System." *Inquiry* 26: 48-61.

_____. 1990. "All-Payer Rate-Setting and the Provision of Hospital Care to the Uninsured: The New Jersey Experience." *Journal of Health Politics, Policy and Law* 15: 815-831.

Salkever, David S., D.M. Steinwachs, and A. Rupp. 1986. "Hospital Cost and Efficiency Under Per Service and Per Case Payment in Maryland: A Tale of the Carrot and the Stick." *Inquiry* 23: 56-66.

Saywell, Robert M., Terrell W. Zolinger, David W. Chu, Charlotte A. MacBeth, and Mary E. Schrist. 1989. "Hospital and Patient Characteristics of Uncompensated Care: Policy Implications." *Journal of Health Politics, Policy and Law* 14(2): 287-307.

Thorpe, Kenneth. 1987. "Does All-Payer Rate-Setting Work? The Case of the New York Prospective Hospital Reimbursement Methodology." *Journal of Health Policies, Policy and Law* 12(3): 391-408.

_____. 1988. "Uncompensated Care Pools and Care to the Uninsured: Lessons From the New York State Prospective Hospital Reimbursement Methodology." *Inquiry* 25: 344-353

Wilensky, Gail R. 1986. "Underwriting the Uninsured: Targeting Providers or Individuals." In Frank A. Sloan, et al., *Uncompensated Care, Rights and Responsibilities*. Baltimore: Johns Hopkins University Press.

Part III

Issues in Policy Implementation

6
Benefit Package Considerations in a State Health Care Plan

David R. Nerenz
Barry M. Zajac
Denise P. Repasky
Patricia D. Williams
Vinod K. Sahney
Henry Ford Health System

When states consider "universal" health plans or plans serving more limited populations, the definition of covered benefits plays a key role in determining the plan's feasibility. In this chapter, considerations about benefit packages, limitations of coverage, cost-sharing characteristics, and covered services are discussed, and a method for estimating program costs is presented.

Types of Benefit Plans

There have traditionally been three main types of health benefit plans: indemnity plans, service benefit plans, and prepaid or capitated plans (Donabedian 1976). Although all three types of plans can provide coverage for the same range of health care services, there have been significant differences among them in how they function and what they ultimately cover.

An indemnity plan is one in which the insured individual pays a regular premium to an insurance company in return for a promise of cash payments should certain defined, insurable events occur. For instance, the insurance company will agree to pay a certain amount for each day of hospitalization, a certain amount for a given outpatient procedure, or a certain amount for a routine office visit.

The agreement is only between the insured individual and the insurance company. The individual is responsible for making payment to the hospital, physician, or other provider for services rendered, and the insurance company provides reimbursement to the insured individual according to the terms of the contract. The amounts of payment are part of the contract, and the individual is responsible for any bills in excess of the agreed upon amounts.

In a service benefit plan, the arrangement is slightly more complex. In return for the premium, the insured individual is entitled to a defined set of health care *services* (that is, days of hospitalization, outpatient treatments, or prescription drugs). The range and level of services are spelled out in the insurance contract, but no fixed dollar amount is assigned to each. To meet its obligation, the insurance company must have another set of agreements in place with providers (hospitals, physicians, and other providers) to actually perform the services that represent the policy's benefits. The insurance company reimburses the providers for services rendered. Providers may or may not bill patients for balances of charges over what the insurance company will pay.

In a prepaid or capitated plan, insured individuals pay a fixed premium, or membership fee, in return for access to virtually all necessary health services provided by members of an organized provider network. Depending on the nature of the relationship between insurer and providers, there may be varying degrees of financial risk on the part of providers. At one extreme, all the members' payments go directly to the provider organization, which in turn is obliged to provide all necessary care and absorb any losses due to excess of expenses over revenues. At another extreme, providers continue to receive fee-for-service or *per diem* payments for services rendered, and the insuring entity takes on the full risk of gain or loss. From the patient perspective, these arrangements are relatively transparent, since patients are not responsible for any payments beyond the premium or membership fee.

These three types of benefit plans have different sets of advantages and disadvantages in terms of administrative overhead, freedom of choice of providers, and sharing of risk among patients/members, insurance companies, and providers. Very broadly speaking, capitation plans usually provide the broadest coverage, most restrictions on choice of providers, least amount of administrative overhead, and least risk of out-of-pocket expenses for the patient. Indemnity plans typically provide much more freedom of choice among providers, but higher administrative costs, more restricted benefits, and higher risk of out-of-pocket expenses in the event of very serious, expensive illness. Service benefit plans share some of the features of indemnity plans, but may have even higher administrative overhead because of the need to process claims information among three parties—the company, the patient, and the provider.

A state-run health care plan could conceivably be based on either of the three basic benefit models, some combination of the three, or perhaps some new model entirely. Choice of model involves some purely technical decisions about how a set of benefits is to be provided most economically, but also involves more value-laden decisions to be made in the political arena. These decisions include: how much choice of providers beneficiaries will have; how much of the current claims-processing infrastructure of existing insurance companies is to be maintained; and how much financial risk is to be the responsibility of the various parties involved in the benefit program.

Benefit Limitations

The design of a health care benefit package must include consideration of what type of limits will or will not be imposed. Some examples of limits in a benefit package include total dollar amount limits, limits on the number of inpatient days, and limits on the number of outpatient visits. Limits are typically imposed to deter overuse of the system by both the patient and provider and to put a ceiling on the financial risk of the insurer. However, due to extreme cases and unique individual circumstances, limits do not *always* control use and costs.

In choosing to impose limits in a state program, policymakers must consider consequences not only in costs, but also in overall utilization patterns and health status. For example, limits on the number of covered outpatient visits could control costs in that area but yield sicker patients upon admission to a hospital. Limits on the number of inpatient days and/or dollar amount limits could lead to earlier discharges and an increased number of outpatient visits. As Donabedian (1976, p. 379) pointed out, "a long list of services is not a sufficient indication of comprehensiveness; stringent limits on the amount of each benefit can cripple the effectiveness of the whole."

In addition, dollar limits on benefits will affect the willingness of providers to render services. Physicians may refuse to offer any services to those with severely restricted benefits without assurance that the patient will be able to pay for any needed care additional to that included in the plan (Donabedian 1976, p. 386). Medicaid, an example of a very comprehensive benefit program in most states, often imposes a strict dollar limit on the amount paid to physicians and hospitals. This type of limit has been shown to lead to patient access problems (Donabedian 1976, p. 264).

Cost-Sharing: Copayments and Deductibles

Health care cost-sharing means patients pay part of the cost of covered services through copayments and/or deductibles. A deductible is an amount of money the beneficiary must spend on health care before eligibility for health insurance benefits begins. Deductibles reduce the claims costs for insurers and may induce patients to avoid seeking care until they have serious symptoms or unless they are confident that they will exceed the deductible amount during the policy period, usually a year. Copayment, or coinsurance, is either a dollar amount or a percentage of a fee that the beneficiary pays at the time of each service. It may create the incentive to avoid prolonged, continuous, or intense care and perhaps to avoid the initiation of care as well (Donabedian 1976).

Cost-sharing helps insurers compensate for "moral hazard," or the tendency for the presence of benefits to change beneficiary behavior in a way that increases use of covered services, by making consumers of care somewhat responsive to its cost. Cost-sharing also reduces the cost of the benefit package and, presumably, the premium. Copayments and deductibles can reduce the administrative costs of claims handling because of fewer claims and because the insurer does not have to pay for any services until the beneficiary spends the deductible amount. Cost-sharing may *increase* costs for the provider, who may have to collect fees from two sources—the patient and a third party (Donabedian 1976).

In a prepaid group practice (PPG), cost-sharing has been shown to affect the use of primary care but have less effect on the types and amounts of other types of office visits used (Cherkin, Grothaus, and Wagner 1989). Copays can reduce the inappropriate use of emergency rooms and unnecessary doctor's office visits. Even very low copayments can effectively prevent unnecessary use (Donabedian 1976; Shapiro, Ware, and Sherbourne 1986). Of course, there is a risk of causing the avoidance of appropriate use among the poor, particularly if copayments are too high, or avoidance of services such as preventive care that are not the result of an acute need. In addition, any delay in seeking care may result in patients being more sick when they do seek care and therefore requiring more intense and expensive treatment (Donabedian 1976).

The effects of cost-sharing measures depend somewhat on the method of provider payment. Since physicians influence the demand for their services and for health care services in general, the incentives *they* face will also affect utilization. To the extent that physicians consider costs to the patient in determining the appropriate course of treatment, patient cost-sharing may affect physician decisionmaking as well (Donabedian 1976). The effects of cost-sharing in a capitated payment situation outside a PPG are not clear, although one might predict that they would depend on the sum of the incentives present. When physicians have an interest in the financial outcome of the plan, they might behave as PPG physicians. Similarly, under a prospective payment system for hospital inpatient care, patient incentives may be immaterial once the patient is hospitalized.

Cost-sharing has other characteristics. A given deductible or copayment amount will have a greater impact on someone with a lower income than on someone with a higher income in terms of percentage of income spent. Similarly, the burden of copays is obviously greater on the ill. These redistributive effects, to use Donabedian's term, are the opposite of those we might endorse, if we would endorse any. When deductibles and copayments are substantial and/or when coverage is not comprehensive, total out-of-pocket expenditures by beneficiaries can be limited to a maximum dollar amount or a percentage of income by a catastrophic coverage provision. This would prevent financial ruin for the families that have a single or series of major medical events, the copayments amounts or uncovered expenses of which they would otherwise be unable to pay (Donabedian 1976).

Any discussion of appropriateness of use presumes that what is appropriate can be satisfactorily defined, which is not necessarily the case. Most studies of the effects of these incentives measure use rates relative to another group. When health risk or health status is the criterion instead, among adults the presence of cost-sharing mechanisms has a negative effect only for the sick and particularly the sick poor (Brook et al. 1983). Children's health has not been found to be affected by the presence of cost-sharing when total out-of-pocket spending is limited to a relatively small amount (Valdez et al. 1985).

The distribution of cost-sharing across a benefit package will influence the mix of services used, particularly in a fee-for-service payment environment. Even very small cost-sharing connected with ambulatory services is associated with lower use of these services and a high rate of hospitalizations among the poor, so that any cost savings on the ambulatory side may be overcome on the inpatient side (Roemer et al. 1975). This type of manipulation of preferences may be helpful if the insurer wishes to encourage certain types of services it feels are relatively economical and/or effective, or to avoid services that may be the opposite. If this were to be done effectively, it would probably require the constant monitoring of the cost and effectiveness of various therapies, settings, and types of providers to assure the most appropriate ones are encouraged, and periodic adjustments to the cost-sharing mechanism. Such a program would probably not be necessary in a PPG, where the most cost-effective therapies are likely to be sought and utilized anyway. Prepaid group practices tend to provide more preventive care and have lower rates of hospitalization (Manning et al. 1984).

Determining Covered Services

The services covered by a benefit package will influence the cost, health benefit, and acceptability to beneficiaries and providers of the health care program. This section will discuss issues surrounding the overall design of the coverage and particular benefits.

There are three main goals in designing a state health care program: to provide adequate access to services for the target population and encourage the appropriate utilization of them; to ensure that the quality of the care received is adequate; and to do so in the most economical way possible. These goals are not independent but interrelated, and the first two may conflict with the last. The resolution of this conflict is not objective or scientific, but political. The determination of what is adequate access and appropriate use is made in the public policy arena, in a context of cost, moderated by the concern with quality.

Access is achieved by having needed services available, in an acceptable way, at an acceptable cost, and within an acceptable distance and time (Penchansky and Thomas 1981). What is "needed" is a matter for debate, but what consumers demand or perceive to be needed must be considered. Acceptability is also a flexible concept that must consider costs (both to society and the consumer), quality, and equity. The criteria by which a particular subpopulation should accept or be found to require a different standard of access from others need to be identified and examined. The payment and participation rates of providers and their geographic distribution will affect access. What benefits are covered and at what cost to the consumer are issues that will affect the consumer's perception of access, which will in some cases affect care-seeking.

Appropriateness of use of health care services can be measured by health outcomes such as infant mortality rates, life expectancy, disability days, and quality-adjusted life years (QALY). Of course, these outcomes are affected by other factors such as the quality of the services, genetics, lifestyle, age, the environment, socioeconomic status, and public health measures, so their value in evaluating health care itself is limited. We know that insurance coverage increases use of health care services, especially among the poor and the sick poor (Davis and Rowland 1983;

Newachek 1988; Wilensky and Berk 1983), although the determination of an appropriate use rate or set of use rates remains normative.

Restricting Use

Plan features restricting use are intended to reduce wasteful or harmful care and control costs. A benefit package can be designed to limit the use of some providers, such as chiropractors or podiatrists, or of some modes of care, such as home care or nursing home care. Insurers may use these restrictions to control their costs, which allows them to maintain competitive prices, market shares, and acceptable margins. This also has the effect of creating and/or maintaining monopoly power and markets for some providers and types of care at the expense of others.

The abhorrence of the idea of rationing health care by ability to pay is one reason for the interest in the financing of health care services for those now uninsured. This interest results from the evolving notion of health care as a right rather than a market good (Callahan 1988; Reinhardt 1986). Credible proposals to make rationing on the basis of age an explicit public policy have been made (Callahan 1987; Aaron and Schwartz 1984) and public debate has begun, but resolution of this issue does not seem near by any means.

The effect of the breadth and depth of the benefit package, or its comprehensiveness, on demand for and use of services is important. If the package is not broad enough (i.e., doesn't have a wide spectrum of covered benefits), it will not encourage efficiency and the types and amounts of use that will maximize the beneficiary's health, well-being, and productivity. There will be a tendency, on the part of providers and beneficiaries, to utilize covered services and avoid services not covered, even if the covered services are inefficient or less effective substitutes for the preferred therapies. This issue is probably more important to states than to private insurers because the states are traditionally responsible for supporting the disabled and medically indigent. Also, if the plan does not protect participants and providers from financial ruin in the event of illness or injury, no matter how catastrophic, it will not be doing what health insurance in its most basic form is supposed to do.

One problem with offering a broad benefit package is that, as costs rise, there is financial pressure to reduce the number of people covered.

This is because the total program costs equal the price of the services offered times the number of services delivered. As costs of the Medicaid benefit package have increased, for instance, most states have adjusted eligibility requirements so those benefits are provided to a population small enough not to exceed budget limitations.

Oregon is trying to reverse this process by limiting the benefits they provide to a predetermined population (Beck, Joseph, and Hager 1990). They have attempted to determine an appropriate and acceptable benefit package by prioritizing covered services according to the expressed preferences of state residents. Through a series of 50 meetings held around the state, over 1,000 residents learned about and expressed their preferences with regard to different therapy options for diseases and their outcomes (Crawshaw et al. 1985). The results of these meetings were tabulated by computer to generate a list of services that could be covered, from highest to lowest priority.

Once this list is finalized, the state legislature intends to determine the cost of coverage for the population they will cover and, using budgetary constraints, to draw a line through the list, which will then define the extent of the benefit package (Beck, Joseph, and Hager 1990). While this process has not cleared all of its administrative hurdles— most important, the receipt of a waiver from the Health Care Financing Administration so it can continue to receive federal contributions to its Medicaid program costs—it represents an innovative and important step toward the rationalization of health care benefits package and program design.

Specific Benefits

Vision and Dental Care

Vision and dental care benefits are often omitted from health care plans to cut costs, on the assumption that their absence will have little or no impact on the general health of the patient. The importance and value of these benefits may not be appreciated. "People seldom die for lack of dental care, but the quality of their lives can be compromised by lack of appropriate care" ("Dental Coverage Affects Usage, Expenditures"

1989). Another reason these benefits are absent from most health care benefit packages is that vision and dental care costs are largely foreseeable and can be planned for (Bell 1980).

The results of partial coverage or no coverage of vision care under a universal health plan will not impact the entire population. However, in design of a universal plan, the fact that half of the population in the United States wears corrective prescription lenses must be taken into consideration ("Vision Care Plans" 1981). For those persons who are unable to afford corrective lenses, partial coverage or a lack of coverage may result in going without glasses or postponement of needed exams, and thus the eye condition may worsen. On the other hand, inclusion of vision care in a universal plan can yield important benefits. The Rand Health Insurance Experiment demonstrated that free vision care resulted in improved vision by increasing the frequency of eye examinations and lens purchase. It is probable that the increased visit rate on the free care plan resulted in increased detection of diseases (Lurie et al. 1989).

In the design of a universal health care plan, the question of covering dental care is difficult. "Dental care may be assumed to have maintained its traditional positive relation to income because it has been regarded by individuals and by society as a more discretionary item, more akin to a luxury than a necessity" (Donabedian 1976, p. 24-25).

Dental plans in general are purchased separately from health insurance plans. The need for dental care is usually predictable and ongoing, rather than episodic like acute health care. According to the American Dental Association, dental benefits differ from medical plans in that dental disease is preventable; early intervention is most efficient and least costly; and the need for care is ongoing and universal ("Coalition, ADA Set Standards for Dental Plans" 1989).

Both dental and vision care are benefits that can be excluded from a health insurance plan with little or no impact on an indicator such as mortality, but could have significant impact on health status/quality of life. However, it may be more cost-efficient to include preventive services in both dental and vision care, thus preventing more expensive treatment in the long term. While health benefits result from including these services in a health care benefit package, the relationship between the benefit and the cost to the state, or any purchaser, is not clear.

Mental Health and Substance Abuse

Use of mental health and substance abuse services by employees and dependents is soaring. According to the National Institute of Mental Health, one of every five Americans now needs professional mental health services, where only one in eight needed such professional help in 1960 (Montgomery 1988). The stigma that was once associated with seeing a psychiatrist or psychologist is no longer as apparent today. Thus, an increase in usage of behavioral health services has caused employers and insurers to look more closely at the cost implications of enhancing coverage that presently exists or including such benefits in a current plan.

Along with an increase in usage, there has been a definite increase in health care dollars being spent on these benefits. Mental health and chemical dependency treatment costs are increasing by more than 15 percent each year (George-Perry 1988). Mental health and substance abuse treatment coverage in health insurance plans have typically been for expensive inpatient care. To deter some of these increasing costs, plans are moving towards more and/or better coverage of outpatient treatment in both of these areas (Frabotta 1989). Outpatient care has been shown in some studies to be less expensive in the long term and to have results that are equal if not better than inpatient care. "Rather than spending $6,000 to $8,000 for an inpatient stay, employers may only have to spend $2,000 to $3,000 for a well-structured, medically supervised outpatient program, while keeping the patient on the job" (Frabotta 1989).

Lack of coverage or partial coverage for behavioral health services will not keep people from being seen in the system. Prior to introduction of specific coverage, and even now with insured groups without coverage, alcoholism was sometimes treated under other "surrogate" diagnoses covered by insurance (Morrisey and Jensen 1988). This type of surrogate treatment is seen with both mental health and substance abuse services.

Various studies have shown that benefits such as mental health and substance abuse actually reduce medical care utilization. "The longitudinal pattern of total health care costs illustrates that a marked increase in such costs among individuals with mental health problems can be expected over the 36-month period prior to initiation of treatment. A decrease in total health care can be expected following the start of mental health treatment—even when costs of this treatment are included" (Holder and Blose 1987). A four-year longitudinal analysis of federal employees showed a decline in health care costs after initiation of treatment. After examining the claims of nearly 1,700 treated alcoholics and their families, one study found that, after an increase in costs associated with treatment, cost for many alcoholics eventually declined to a point comparable with the lowest pretreatment levels (Holder and Blose 1986).

The inclusion of such benefits in an insurance plan may decrease total health care costs and be beneficial; however, it may be necessary to implement limits to have some type of control on utilization of these services. The open-ended nature of psychiatric treatment frequency invites continuation of outpatient contact with the therapist far beyond the point of symptom remission (Montgomery 1988).

Prescription Drugs and Contraceptives

Prescription drugs are covered under many health insurance plans with little or no copayment. However, prescription coverage, once viewed as a small investment that brought about large returns, is now being reconsidered, and tighter controls are being implemented. The reason is that the cost of coverage is rising. For many companies, the cost of covering prescription drugs has risen faster than any other component of their health benefits package except mental health and substance abuse treatment (Vibbert 1989). Covering prescription drugs without any type of utilization control mechanism can result in high costs under a universal plan. On the other hand, not covering prescription drugs under this plan may have effects on health. The lack of prescription drug coverage could affect some persons more than others—for example, those below a certain income level who just cannot afford such "extras" as prescription drugs.

In many plans, contraceptives fall under the category of prescription drugs; however, they may be viewed as a separate benefit in the design of a health insurance plan. Many insurance plans are beginning to drop coverage of contraceptives due to the cost that this coverage adds to the premium (Muller 1978). Offering coverage of contraceptives as prescription drugs will add to the cost of a plan in the near term, however, in the long term it may decrease utilization of obstetrical and pediatric health care services.

Experimental Procedures

Treatments and procedures considered experimental are generally exempted, or not covered, by health care plans (Ham 1989). The determination of whether or not something is experimental is made in several ways, but it is common for insurers to follow the example of the Health Care Financing Administration, which makes this determination for the Medicare and Medicaid programs. If exempted, a procedure may be available to those who have the ability and willingness to pay for it out-of-pocket or to those who can find and are eligible for participation in a funded research project that will pay for it. The rationale for not covering these treatments is that their efficacy and safety have not been proven, and their use is not widely accepted. In addition, they tend to be expensive. Since these therapies are not widely available, states should have little problem exempting them from the benefit package. There is not an equity issue since others do not have access either, and there is a cost and quality interest in not covering care until it is shown to be safe and have a useful place in the medical armamentarium.

Transplants

The coverage of organ and tissue transplants has received considerable attention. Both Arizona and Oregon have restricted coverage of transplants for their Medicaid recipients. Considering the high costs and the poor cost-effectiveness of some of these life-saving or sustaining procedures compared to other potential uses of funds, noncoverage may be a rational choice (Durbin 1988). On the other hand, since most private insurance plans cover at least some and usually most of the costs of such procedures, and some transplants may be more cost-effective than the alternative therapies for the afflicted individuals, noncoverage raises equity and discrimination issues (Durbin 1988). In the context of a universal plan, these issues would be less potent because the same coverage would apply to everyone. When participants in the plan are disproportionately of a particular socioeconomic status or racial or ethnic group, special effort may be needed to avoid the appearance or fact of discrimination.

New Technology

One of the effects of a "free market" medical system has been the development of new technologies, especially in the areas of pharmaceuticals, surgical procedures, biotechnology, and imaging. Treatments constantly emerge for conditions previously considered untreatable, and new and innovative treatments replace old (McGregor 1989). This march of technology is a source of both pride and concern. While these technologies are largely responsible for our health care system being seen as the best in the world, they also are a central reason for the tremendous costs and inflation experienced in the health care sector. They also tend to shift resources away from prevention and primary care (Somers 1984). That private insurers generally provide coverage for new technologies only on the basis of efficacy and availability without regard to costs certainly contributes to this dilemma (Ham 1989). While not all of these technologies are as expensive as Positron Emission Tomography or AZT, they all contribute to the health cost spiral (Moloney and Rogers 1979).

When sick, Americans expect access to the latest and most innovative technology, even when its cost outweighs any incremental benefit that may be achieved over the technology it replaces. An example is electronic fetal heart monitoring, which is widely if not routinely used, even though its benefits are unproven (Shy et al. 1990). For this reason, it would be difficult to exclude coverage of new technologies in a comprehensive state benefit package. There are several strategies for controlling the use of these technologies. One approach would be to require prior approval for the use of specified procedures on a case-by-case basis. This could operate similarly to prehospitalization certification programs whereby the payor must approve any nonemergency hospital admission. Copayments and/or deductibles could also be attached to discourage overuse. Still another strategy would put the provider at financial risk for the use of the procedure or technology through a capitated or case-based payment system (Moloney and Rogers 1979). The use of cost-effectiveness analysis remains an untried and potentially potent basis for such allocative decisionmaking (Emery and Schneiderman 1989).

It would be a mistake, however, to take the view that it is only new or high technology that is responsible for an increase in costs of treatments. Increases in the use of existing technology, such as X-ray examinations and laboratory tests, are as likely to be culprits. Strategies to limit the use of technology are best if they apply to any type. Examples could be capitation of case-based payment or broad-utilization review (Moloney and Rogers 1979).

Rehabilitation

After a disabling injury or illness, such as an auto accident or a stroke, patients may be discharged from the hospital without need of continuing medical care but still unable to resume life as before. Although many of these individuals ultimately will be unable to recover fully, they may still be able to lead personally fulfilling and socially productive lives, provided they receive the rehabilitation services required. There are other sources of financing for rehabilitation services. In some states, the no-fault auto insurance program may include this coverage in the event of an auto accident. Workers' compensation insurance provides this coverage for injuries that occur in the workplace. Still, there are circumstances outside of these environments, such as strokes, and accidents other than motor vehicle, when the services necessary to maximize a patient's potential is not accessible due to lack of financing. This is a particularly important issue for states, which, unlike private insurers, are traditionally responsible for the welfare of their citizens, have a potential tax-generating workforce in need of services, and have to pay a proportion of Title XIX program costs of those who remain disabled. If states already have a rehabilitation program in place, the effect of this coverage on its costs should be considered.

Rehabilitation services can be rationed in several ways. A common method is to set a time limit after which services would no longer be covered or a set number of services or amount of dollars allowed. This can be seen as discriminatory against those who, while significant recovery is expected, have injuries that necessitate longer or more intensive rehabilitation. Another way would be to provide coverage for only a specific set of services based on the prognosis, or to make a determination of coverage based on the prognosis and the expected rehabilitation time or expense. Someone whose rehabilitation would take a shorter time and who is expected to make a more complete recovery would have services covered, while others may not. Prognosis accuracy would be important in both of these situations, which may be a problem. Age and social role could also be considered in such decisions.

The costs associated with transplants, new technology, and rehabilitation may be most appropriately managed in the context of a program for catastrophic health care cost protection. These rather extreme sources of high costs are singled out, perhaps because they affect a very small number of people. Chronic disease treatment and intensive care also involve very high expenses, but there is no suggestion that they be excised from the health care package. On the contrary, they are important reasons for having coverage. Efforts to control costs may be more effective and fair through a systemwide approach to efficiency, utilization management, and prevention than by the narrowing of the benefit package at its margins where those with great need are denied and emotional responses and inflammatory press coverage are likely.

Home Health Care

Home health care has become an important low-cost substitute for hospital and nursing home care. Therapies that were once considered strictly inpatient, requiring high levels of nursing skill, have found their way into the realm of home care. Patients can be safely discharged home from the hospital earlier when regular skilled nursing care is available in the home (American Medical Association Council on Scientific Affairs 1990). This can bring considerable cost savings to the payor while improving outcomes (for instance, through the avoidance of nosocomial infections) and patient satisfaction. Additional costs can occur, however, when home care is sought that is not a substitute for other medical care. This is an example of the effect of "moral hazard," because demand seems to come as a result of the provision of coverage. It is not clear in these circumstances whether this demand represents substitution for family care or for impending medical care. If it is a substitute for future hospital care, it may represent a source of additional savings in the long run, rather than a liability.

The use of home health care can be restricted, for instance, by only covering services provided after a hospitalization, and then for a limited time, as Medicare does, and/or by attaching cost-sharing provisions. Requiring prior approval by the payer would be another strategy. Home health care is such a valuable and efficient model of care that its coverage should probably be considered essential to even a basic health plan, even if restrictions are attached.

Durable Medical Equipment

Like home health care, durable medical equipment (DME) is a valuable service for beneficiaries that can reduce the cost of care but has potential for overuse or abuse. By providing respiratory therapy equipment, wheelchairs, walkers, special beds, and appliances, the well-being and quality of life of patients can be enhanced. In some cases, these services represent less intensive treatment methods than would otherwise be employed, and thereby represent a cost savings. When improved comfort and well-being improves health and avoids the need for other forms of care, additional savings may accrue, although this has not been quantified. The downside is that these services may be used unnecessarily just because they are available, or as substitutes for goods or services that would have otherwise been paid for out-of-pocket. Cost-sharing may also be applied here, as well as utilization management or risk-assumption by the provider.

Estimating Costs of a State Health Care Program

With the above considerations in mind, estimates of costs for a benefit package to be offered under a state-sponsored plan can be generated. Estimates are useful for considering the effects of variations in a benefit package and other elements of a program on its overall costs. As an example, we estimated the cost of covering Michigan residents under 65 with a comprehensive package for implementation in 1990 or 1991.

Data Sources

One way to estimate costs would be to estimate utilization rates based on known averages and apply a per-service cost model to calculate overall costs. This requires realistic estimates of costs, which are difficult to obtain, and assumes that patterns of use will not be affected by a new program. Another way to estimate costs would be to use known per-patient costs and apply them to the target population.

We found data on the latter to be readily available through a state health maintenance organization (HMO) regulating agency. Few non-HMO plans provide a comprehensive set of benefits, particularly for outpatient care and preventive services. HMO plans provide the best and most current data on the costs of this type of package.

While Medicaid also offers a comprehensive benefit package, its unique demographics, the large concentration of elderly and disabled, possible differences in utilization (for example, lower use of services because of access problems), lack of controls on utilization, and unrealistic provider payment make its experience a poor basis for cost projections to the whole population.

We estimate the costs of benefits with data from the 1989 rate filing of Blue Care Network (BCN), Michigan's second largest HMO. This HMO's data were used because:

1. This large HMO has subscribers throughout most of Michigan. Its cost experience may be more typical of what could be expected under a statewide plan than that of HMOs that serve a limited geographic area or have very small enrollments.
2. The division of the plan into geographically defined subunits allows a comparison of costs of care in different areas of the state.
3. Comparisons of BCN and other HMOs showed that it is typical in having neither the highest nor lowest per-member per-month (PMPM) costs.
4. These data reflect managed care delivery as proposed for the Michigan plan. BCN is typical of the sorts of plans offered if consumers are

allowed to choose from among several certified health care plans. As a network-model HMO, Blue Care Network does not have all the cost-containment features of staff- or group-model HMOs, but has some not found in purely fee-for-service plans. Its experience, therefore, is a middle ground between the most and least efficient financing and delivery system models.

5. BCN subscribers are diverse. The plan is not restricted to white- or blue-collar employees, and most age and economic groups are represented.

The benefit package used is summarized in Table 1. Using specific health plan data requires caution. Some caveats and issues we considered are:

1. Projections were based on 1988 data. Utilization rates and costs per unit of service—or the data itself—may have been anomalous for some reason that year. More precise forecasts using these data would consider the relationship of the 1988 data to both 1987 and 1989.

2. We did not usually have information on exactly what costs are reflected in the costs per unit of service that are a part of the monthly cost estimate. These are provider costs that may change in a number of unpredictable ways under a state health plan. There might be reductions in inpatient care costs due to eliminating uncompensated care, reduced billing costs, or lowered malpractice costs.

3. Dental and vision care costs do not come from Blue Care Network. The costs of dental coverage are from 1988 information for Blue Cross-Blue Shield. The costs of vision coverage are from the 1988 rate filing of Comprehensive Health Services of Detroit, a Detroit HMO. In both cases the costs represent an approximation of a median cost estimate—neither the highest nor lowest cost for this benefit.

4. The average cost figure shown for the benefit package is an unweighted average of the costs of these benefits from six BCN regional plans. The average was not weighted for the size of the enrolled population because the largest plan occasionally had specific benefit costs that were unusually high or low when compared to either the other Blue Care Network plans or other HMO rate filing information.

Table 1
Summary of Benefit Cost Findings

Benefit	Copay	1989 costs (PMPM)*
Inpatient		
Hospital charges (unlimited days, semi-private room, and specialized units)		$23.82
Professional services		8.30
Outpatient		
Office visits (including preventive, urgent and specialist care)	$5.00	16.87
Diagnostic services (X-ray and lab work)		7.52
Outpatient surgery		4.31
Allergy testing/serum	50%	0.15
Other outpatient services	$5.00	1.49
Reproductive health		
Adult sterilizations	50%	0.15
Elective terminations	50%	0.07
Mental health		
Inpatient mental health		1.30
Inpatient substance abuse	50%	0.80
Outpatient mental health	50%	1.42
Outpatient substance abuse	50%	0.53
Emergency care		
Emergency care	$25.00	2.71
Ambulance		0.47
Other		
Skilled nursing facility (up to 45 days)		0.08
Home health agency	$5.00	0.35
Durable medical equipment	20%	0.27
Pharmacy (including needles, syringes and birth control)	$3.00	9.51
Other services		1.05
Dental		10.51
Vision		1.77
Benefit total		**$93.48**
Reinsurance		1.15
Administration and retention (16%)		15.14
TOTAL		**$109.77**

*per member per month.

An unweighted average seemed more likely to yield a *conservative* estimate of the future cost of benefits.

5. Not all benefits were offered in all plans—in most cases because services were offered under one of the other benefit categories (for example, urgent care could have been a separate category or included under an office visit category). Most of these differences are resolved by combining the categories into a single benefit, others by leaving zeroes out of average cost calculations. The result is an average that is slightly higher (or more conservative) than the average that would have been calculated from each of the plans' total costs.

Adjustment in Estimates to Project Costs for a State Program

Before data from an existing plan are used to project costs for a state program, it is necessary to determine if there is a selection bias present in the plan membership that would affect cost projections. The membership of the plan used to model costs must match the population to be covered by a new program in factors that predict utilization and costs or be adjusted to compensate for differences. Table 2 summarizes demographic differences between the 1988 BCN enrolled population and the 1990 projections for the entire State of Michigan. There are only minor differences in the age and gender composition of the populations.

Based on the small differences between the BCN and Michigan populations, no adjustment appeared necessary. Variations seem to have effects on health care costs that would balance each other. BCN has more women of childbearing age and adults between 55 and 64 (higher costs), but also more children (lower costs). Therefore, based on the age and sex distributions of its membership, this plan seemed to be a reasonable basis for projecting overall costs for the state of a universal plan.

Variation in Costs by Region of the State

An important issue to be worked out during discussion of a state plan is the extent to which the state will wish to adjust its contribution on the basis of geographical variation in costs. Our estimate for all of

Table 2
Comparing State and HMO Populations

Age	Michigan*			Blue Care Network**		
	Total	Male (percent)	Female	Total	Male (percent)	Female
0–19	33.5	17.1	16.4	37.9	19.3	18.6
20–24	9.1	4.7	4.4	7.2	3.2	4.0
25–34	19.5	9.6	9.9	19.6	8.9	10.7
35–44	17.0	8.4	8.6	18.1	8.9	9.2
45–54	11.3	5.5	5.8	10.1	5.1	5.0
55–64	9.6	4.6	5.1	6.8	3.3	3.5

*Michigan population data were obtained from the Michigan Department of Management and Budget and represent the entire population of Michigan projected for 1990. This includes individuals who are currently insured through their employers, as well as individuals covered on nongroup plans, public programs such as Medicaid, or without any health insurance.

**Blue Care Network covers primarily small-, medium- and large-group business with perhaps 1 to 3 percent nongroup business in 1988.

Michigan would be reasonable if a single, statewide plan were implemented. If, however, individuals were allowed to choose from among several plans that may serve limited areas, state contributions or allowable premiums *may* be adjusted for regional variation in costs.

In a previous analysis we found rates for a large commercial insurer varied by area within Michigan as shown in Table 3. There was much less cost variation between BCN regions, and the Southeast region (Detroit and its suburbs) did not have the highest projected costs. Since costs of coverage are a function of several factors, including characteristics of the enrolled population, use rates, costs per unit of service, and costs of plan administration, it is difficult to do further analysis of cost variations within the state for a universal plan until more specific information is available. It may be that the lower costs of benefits in areas such as the Upper Peninsula may be balanced by higher administrative costs there due to low population density.

Table 3
Regional Variations in Premiums

Area	Rate multiplier
Upper Peninsula, some Northern Lower	1.00
"Outstate" Lower Peninsula	1.07
Lansing, Kalamazoo, "Downriver" areas	1.14
Macomb, Oakland, Washtenaw counties (suburban Detroit)	1.25
Wayne County (includes City of Detroit)	1.38

Costs of Individual and Family Coverage

Our best current estimate is that a figure of approximately $110 per month per person would be a reasonable projection of the 1989 costs of a comprehensive health care plan for a large group with demographics like those of the Michigan population (including children, not including individuals over 65). Projected premiums for single adults and families are determined by applying multipliers to the average PMPM cost according to how costs are to be distributed across these groups. An example is shown in Table 4.

Table 4
Determining Premiums for Beneficiary Groups

Group	Multiplier	Premium
Base (Average PMPM)		=$109.77
Single adult	=Base x 1.25	=$137.21
Couple	=Base x 2.88	=$316.14
Family	=Base x 3.26	=$357.85

Precision of Cost Estimates

The accuracy of estimates of the costs of coverage for a proposed program depends on several factors for which our data were incomplete:

- health status and utilization patterns of group to be covered
- delivery system(s) in which care is to be provided
- whether payment will be based on premiums charged by insurers, including all administrative expenses, or a reduced premium which does not allow recovery of all insurer costs, or a rate pegged more closely to the costs of providing care
- whether providers will be reimbursed on a charge basis, an "allowable fee" basis, a capitation basis, or some sort of partial recovery basis less than full costs
- additional cost-containment features that may be built into the design of the plan.

There are some clear tradeoffs between costs of coverage, extent of coverage, and the administrative and delivery system structures associated with any plan. In our example, $110 per-person per-month can purchase very extensive coverage in most areas of the state under circumstances exemplified by Blue Care Network. It will purchase much less extensive coverage in a high-cost area of the state and/or under plans with higher administrative costs (for example, individual or small-group coverage).

Finally, it must be considered that implementation of a state plan may itself affect costs. Here are some ways that the plan can distort its own costs.

1. As uninsured individuals become covered, a short increase in demand for services could occur, resulting in higher-than-normal costs due to "pent-up" demand.
2. The burst of demand may meet some serious shortages of health care providers, particularly nurses in acute-care settings and physicians in areas that are currently underserved. Not all individuals seeking care and covered by the state plan will be able to get it quickly. The increase in use will therefore be moderated in the near term, but will last as long as there continues to be a demand backlog.
3. If features of a state plan create a significant restriction on physician incomes, an exodus of physicians may occur if it is not countered by other changes making practice in the state more desirable. Any migration will affect access to care and in turn program costs and the program's ability to meet its objectives.

There are other possible effects of implementation that are impossible to predict with any certainty until the features of a plan are made more specific. As discussion and planning move forward, it will be possible to adjust cost estimates to reflect how plan features relate to utilization and costs per unit of service.

It is difficult to accurately predict how changes in some of these factors will affect costs of providing care. Our estimates of the costs of providing services under managed care conditions in the Blue Care Network environment are based on patterns of use and costs of providing services specific to BCN. If conditions change drastically under a state plan, simple linear projections of past trends to future costs, while they may be the best estimates available, will be subject to more than the usual amount of error. The purpose of these analyses is to roughly estimate the effects of various benefit combinations on the overall program costs to a state. They are not intended to be the basis for budgeting. As plans move closer to implementation, more precise and actuarially sound cost calculations must be performed.

Conclusion

The design of a benefit package will affect every aspect of a program: its success at meeting its health and social objectives, such as financial equity for providers, income redistribution, and improvement in the health status of target populations; its costs and their distribution between payors, patients, and providers; and (therefore and inevitably) its political viability. A well-conceived benefit package can remove ambiguity about the goals of a program and its expected costs and advantages.

Accomplishing this requires that knowledge of the effects of benefit features be injected into a process of values clarification about program goals that is essentially political. Priority-setting with regard to beneficiaries (providers, payors, and patients), and benefits (considering implicit rationing from restricted coverage) can be assisted by the provision of information about the costs and effects of specific benefit changes.

References

Aaron, H. J. and William B. Schwartz. 1984. *The Painful Prescription: Rationing Hospital Care*. Washington, DC: The Brookings Institution.

American Medical Association Council on Scientific Affairs. 1990. "Home Care in the 1990s," *Journal of the American Medical Association* 263(9): 1241-44 (March 2).

Beck, Melinda, Nadine Joseph, and Mary Hager. 1990. "Not Enough for All: Oregon Experiments with Rationing Health Care," *Newsweek* (May 14): 53-55.

Bell, Donald R. 1980. "Dental and Vision Care Benefits in Health Insurance Plans," *Monthly Labor Review* 103(6): 22-26.

Brook, Robert H., John E. Ware, William H. Rogers, Emmett B. Keeler, Allyson R. Davies, Cathy A. Donald, George A. Goldberg, Kathleen N. Lohr, Patricia C. Masthay, and Joseph P. Newhouse. 1983. "Does Free Care Improve Adults' Health?," *New England Journal of Medicine* 309(23): 1426-34.

Callahan, Daniel. 1988. "Meeting Needs and Rationing Care," *Law, Medicine and Health Care* 16(3-4): 261-66.

_____. 1987. *Setting Limits: Medical Goals in an Aging Society*. NY: Simon & Schuster.

Cherkin, Daniel C., Louis Grothaus, and Edward H. Wagner. 1989. "The Effect of Office Visit Copayments on Utilization in a Health Maintenance Organization," *Medical Care* 27(7): 669-79.

"Coalition, ADA Set Standards For Dental Plans." 1989. *Employee Benefit Plan Review* (May): 14-16.

Crawshaw, Ralph, Michael Garland, Brian Hines, and Caroline Lobitz. 1985. "Oregon Health Decisions: An Experiment in Community Consent," *Journal of the American Medical Association* 254(22): 3213-16.

Davis, K. and D. Rowland. 1983. "Uninsured and Underserved: Inequities in Health Care in the United States," *Milbank Memorial Fund Quarterly* 61: 149-76.

"Dental Coverage Affects Usage, Expenditures." 1989. *Employee Benefit Plan Review* (May): 17-19.

Donabedian, Avedis. 1976. *Benefits in Medical Care Programs*. Cambridge, MA: Harvard University Press.

Durbin, Meg. 1988. "Bone Marrow Transplantation: Economic, Ethical, and Social Issues," *Pediatrics* 82(5): 774-83.

Emery, Danielle Dolenc and Lawrence J. Schneiderman. 1989. "Cost-Effectiveness Analysis in Health Care," *Hastings Center Report* (July/August): 8-13.

Frabotta, Judith. 1989. "How to Weigh Drug Treatment Options," *Business and Health* 7(2): 37-38.

George-Perry, Sharon. 1988. "Easing the Costs of Mental Health Benefits," *Personnel Administrator* 33(11): 62-67.

Ham, Faith Lyman. 1989. "How Insurers Decide to Cover Technology," *Business & Health* (November): 32-34.

Holder, Harold D. and James O. Blose. 1987. "Changes in Health Care Costs and Utilization Associated With Mental Health Treatment," *Hospital and Community Psychiatry* 38(10):1070-75.

_____. 1986. "Alcoholism Treatment and Total Health Care Utilization and Costs," *Journal of the American Medical Association* 256(11): 1456-60.

Lurie, Nicole, Caren J. Kamberg, Robert H. Brook, Emmett B. Keeler, and Joseph P. Newhouse. 1989. "How Free Care Improved Vision in the Health Insurance Experiment," *American Journal of Public Health* 79(5): 640-42.

Manning, Willard G., Arleen Leibowitz, George A. Goldberg, William H. Rogers, and Joseph P. Newhouse. 1984. "A Controlled Trial of the Effect of a Prepaid Group Practice on the Use of Services," *New England Journal of Medicine* 310(23): 1505-10.

McGregor, Maurice. 1989. "Technology and the Allocation of Resources," *New England Journal of Medicine* 320(2): 118-20.

Moloney, Thomas W. and David E. Rogers. 1979. "Medical Technology—A Different View of the Contentious Debate Over Costs," *New England Journal of Medicine* 301(26): 1413-19.

Montgomery, John S. 1988. "Shrink Mental Health Care Costs," *Personnel Journal* 67(5): 86-91.

Morrisey, M.A. and G.A. Jensen. 1988. "Employer-Sponsored Insurance Coverage for Alcoholism and Drug-Abuse Treatments," *Journal of Studies on Alcohol* 49(5): 456-61.

Muller, Charlotte F. 1978. "Insurance Coverage of Abortion, Contraception & Sterilization," *Family Planning Perspectives* 10(12): 71-77.

Newachek, P.W. 1988. "Access to Ambulatory Care for Poor Persons," *Health Services Research* 23: 401-19.

Penchansky, R. and William J. Thomas. 1981. "The Concept of Access: Definition and Relation to Consumer Satisfaction," *Medical Care* 19: 127-39.

Reinhardt, Uwe E. 1986. "Rationing the Health-Care Surplus: An American Tragedy," *Nursing Economics* 4(3): 101-8.

Roemer, Milton I., Carl E. Hopkins, Lockwood Carr, and Foline Gartside. 1975. "Copayments for Ambulatory Care: Penny-Wise and Pound-Foolish," *Medical Care* 13(6): 457-66.

Scitovsky, Anne A. 1985. "Changes in the Costs of Treatment of Selected Illnesses, 1971-1981," *Medical Care* 23(12): 1345-57.

Shapiro, Martin F., John E. Ware, Jr., and Cathy Donald Sherbourne. 1986. "Effects of Cost Sharing on Seeking Care for Serious and Minor Symptoms: Results of a Randomized Trial," *Annals of Internal Medicine* 104(2): 246-51.

Shy, Kirkwood K., David Luthy, Forrest Bennett, Michael Whitfield, Eric B. Larson, Gerald van Belle, James P. Hughes, Judith A. Wilson, and Morton A. Stenchever. 1990. "The Effects of Electronic Fetal-Heart-Rate Monitoring, as Compared with Periodic Auscultation, on the Neurologic Development of Premature Infants," *New England Journal of Medicine* 322(9): 588-93.

Somers, Anne R. 1984. "Why Not Try Preventing Illness as a Way of Controlling Medicare Costs?" *New England Journal of Medicine* 311(13): 853-56.

Valdez, R. Burciaga, Robert H. Brook, William H. Rogers, John E. Ware, Emmett B. Keeler, Cathy A. Sherbourne, Kathleen N. Lohr, George A. Goldberg, Patricia Camp, and Joseph P. Newhouse. 1985. "Consequences of Cost Sharing for Children's Health," *Pediatrics* 75(5): 952-61.

Vibbert, Spencer. 1989. "How to Restrain Ballooning Drug Benefit Costs," *Business & Health* 7(4): 39-46.

"Vision Care Plans." 1981. *Personnel Journal* 60(10): 760,762.

Wilensky, G.R. and M. Berk. 1983. "Poor, Sick, and Uninsured," *Health Affairs* 2: 91-95.

7

Public Financing Approaches to Improve Access to Health Care

Alternative Revenue Sources

John E. Anderson
University of Nebraska

Improved health care access is not free. States wishing to provide improved access must address the question of how to pay the added costs involved. If the cost of improved access is to be funded through a general tax mechanism, the questions to be asked are: What tax sources may be tapped and what revenues may be reasonably expected? In addition, it is important to question both the equity and efficiency aspects of the proposed tax sources of funding. We need to know both who will pay the tax and how the tax will affect economic decisions and the allocation of resources. The goal of tax policy is to design tax mechanisms that are fair and nondistortionary.

Tax policy changes which could fund health care access are identified in this chapter for each of the typical state's major taxes—sales and excise taxes, personal income or payroll taxes, and business taxes. Each tax is defined by its base (what is taxed) and its rate (how much is taxed). We will consider changes in the rate of taxation and in the definition of the tax base, which could be used to generate revenue for improving access to health care. As part of the base change proposals, we will consider elimination of some specific tax expenditures—exemptions or deductions—as potential revenue sources.[1]

Sales and Excise Tax Sources

State and local governments rely on sales and excise taxes for a substantial portion of their own-source revenue. The general sales tax accounts for about 14 percent of state-local general revenue in the United

States. The percentage ranges from a high of 29 percent in Washington State and 25 percent in Tennessee to a low of 7 percent in Vermont.[2] There are also five states without a general sales tax: New Hampshire, Delaware, Montana, Oregon, and Alaska. In addition to the state sales tax, many states permit local sales taxes, making the combined state-local sales tax rate higher. The highest combined rate is that of New York City—8.25 percent.

With this reliance on the general sales tax, it is natural to ask whether improved access to health care could be funded through increased general sales taxes. There are two basic ways to increase the sales tax. One is to raise the tax rate, say, from a state's current 5 percent to 6 percent or 7 percent. The other is to broaden the tax base, taxing more goods or services than the tax is currently levied against. We will discuss each of these possibilities in turn.

Sales Tax Rate Change

A sales tax rate increase will raise revenue, the precise amount depending upon the size of the tax base. As an example, consider the Michigan sales tax at its current rate of 4 percent. The sales tax generates $2.6 billion (FY89 DMB estimate) in revenue. Including the state use tax puts the total at $3 billion.[3] The combined tax base is therefore $75 billion ($3 billion divided by .04). Hence, a 1 percent increase in the tax will generate $750 million in revenue. This estimate overstates the revenue that will be generated, however, since as prices rise due to the higher tax, fewer goods will be demanded, reducing the tax base. The precise reduction in the tax base will depend upon the elasticity of demand for those commodities being taxed.

One potential problem in raising a state sales tax rate is the border effect, when neighboring states have substantially lower tax rates. Taxable economic activity may be shifted to the lower tax state when the potential tax saving is large enough to cover the added expense of moving the transaction site.

Sales Tax Base Changes

A direct way to increase general sales tax revenue is to tax goods or services not currently taxed. Most states exempt food and prescription drugs from the general sales tax for equity reasons—to make the sales tax less regressive. (A tax is regressive when the portion of income paid in tax falls as income rises and progressive when the opposite holds.) Other common exemptions designed to relieve the regressivity of the sales tax are those for clothing or household gas/electric. While some revenue could be gained by eliminating these exemptions, they are a necessary part of the sales tax base definition intended to reduce the regressiveness of the tax.

Tax General Services

The major way to change the sales tax base is to extend the tax to services. Presently, the sales tax applies to commodities but not to services (at least not to very many services). Economists have suggested that this differential treatment of commodities and services causes distortions in the economy's allocation of resources between the two. There is a clear incentive to shift resources into services and away from commodities to avoid the tax. For example, the present system taxes a new shirt purchased at a retail store, but exempts the laundering of the shirt from taxation. Why should the tax system distort the decision on whether to purchase a new shirt or launder old shirts? On efficiency grounds, we would like the tax system to be neutral, not affecting such decisions. If we were to broaden the base of the sales tax to include services, we could either reduce the tax rate and collect the same revenues or make available additional revenues. As an example, if the State of Michigan were to tax all services, an additional $1 billion in revenue would be generated at the state's present 4 percent tax rate.[4] The largest category of services is health services, taxation of which would generate $479.8 million annually in Michigan.

Such a change in the tax will, of course, generate criticism, as Florida's recent experience has clearly illustrated (Hellerstein 1988). Florida's attempt to broaden the state sales tax to include services was vigorously opposed by advertising firms whose products would have been subjected to the tax. Despite the potential for political opposition, the notion of taxing services deserves careful consideration.[5]

The taxation of health care services would have the effect of increasing the price of such services and reducing the equilibrium quantity of the services. Estimates of the elasticity of demand for hospital care services are in the range of 0.7 or less, which indicates that consumers are not very sensitive to price changes. In addition, if the supply of health care services is relatively elastic (responsive to price changes), the incidence of the tax on health care services would be borne mostly by the consumers of the care, not the producers. Improved access to health care financed in this way would raise the price of care for *all* in order to provide access for *some*.

The distributional effects of broadening the sales tax base to include health-related services can be investigated using recent research on the sales tax base. Bohm and Craig (1987) have simulated service-sector expenditures as a percentage of income for a number of services, including several health-related services. Their estimates of the distribution of expenditures indicate that extending the sales tax to health-related services will be regressive.[6] Consumption expenditures as a percent of income fall as income rises. Consequently, applying the sales tax to these services will disproportionately fall on the poor.

This problem could be partially corrected by applying a refundable credit on the state income tax for sales taxes paid. The income tax credit could be designed to phase out with income, relieving the regressivity of the sales tax for low income levels. Net revenue from the sales tax on services less the income tax credit for sales tax paid on health services could then be used to fund improved access to health care.

Table 1 provides aggregate U.S. data on several alternative sales tax bases. The first alternative is to tax consumption, less expenditures on food and all services. This results in a narrow tax base, $998.3 billion, similar to the present tax base used by most states. A somewhat broader tax base could be constructed by taxing consumption less expenditures on food, housing, medical care and household gas and electric. The resulting tax base is $1,784.1 billion, or a tax base about 1.79 times larger than the present tax base. An even broader tax base to consider would be taxing consumption less expenditures on housing and medical care. In that case, the tax base is $2,467.5 billion, a tax base 2.47 times larger than the present tax base. These data indicate that substantially more revenue can be generated from the sales tax by including services. These figures are broadly suggestive of the potential revenues that would follow from sales tax base-broadening at the state level, although regional differences in consumption patterns would affect the revenues involved.

Table 1
Alternate Sales Tax Bases, 1989

	$ billions
Personal income	4,396.2
Disposable personal income	3,744.5
Personal consumption	3,437.9
Consumption expenditures	
Food	588.6
Clothing	198.5
Services	1,851.0
Housing	527.5
Medical care	442.9
Gas and electric	94.8
Alternate tax bases	
1. Consumption less expenditures on food and all services	998.3
2. Consumption less expenditures on food, housing, medical care, and household gas and electric	1,784.1
3. Consumption less expenditures on housing and medical care	2,467.5

SOURCE: U.S. Department of Commerce, *Survey of Current Business*, July 1989, pp. 50, 51.

Tax Amusements and Recreation Services

By extending the sales tax to amusements and recreation services, additional revenue could be generated. This base-broadening would apply the state sales tax to theater and athletic tickets and other such recreation or amusement admission charges. The distributional consequences of such taxation are not known with precision. While theater ticket taxation would probably fall on the wealthy, athletic contest ticket admission taxation would probably affect lower-income consumers. Recent work by Blair, Giarratani, and Spiro (1987) indicates that an amusement tax may not be shifted to ticket purchasers (through higher ticket prices) at all in the case of sports franchises, may only be shifted partially in the case of nonprofit concert and theater series, and is only partially shifted in the long run for movie theaters. Overall, we do not know how the tax would be borne by low-income residents relative to high-income residents of a state, but this work indicates only partial shifting of the tax burden.

Tax Interstate Sales

Taxing interstate sales would generate additional revenue. Currently, state sales taxes typically apply to those businesses with a tax nexus in the state, i.e., retail outlets in the state. As a result, national retailers such as L.L. Bean who do not have such nexus in the state do not collect sales or use tax on purchases by customers in the state. Hence, present tax administration and policy favors purchase of a shirt from the L.L. Bean catalog over purchase of the same shirt from a local department store.[7] Such differential tax treatment of the same commodity is inefficient, encouraging tax avoidance activity, and should be remedied. There are substantial administrative difficulties in taxing interstate sales, although these problems have been a topic of discussion at the state and national levels for several years and expedient solutions are being formulated.[8]

The incidence of such a tax is likely to be the same as that for the sales tax on intrastate sales. There is no particular reason to believe that consumers ordering from retailers outside a given state differ substantially from those purchasing goods from retailers within that state. To the extent that some of the interstate sales are attributed to upscale catalog retailers, the incidence may be somewhat more progressive than the normal sales tax.

Cigarette Excise Tax Rate Change[9]

States vary widely in their taxation of cigarettes. Table 2 illustrates the current rate of taxation in the states, varying from a low of $.02 per package in North Carolina to a high of $.40 per package in Connecticut. The southern tobacco-producing states tend to have very low rates of taxation; for example, the tax is $.03 in Kentucky and $0.025 in Virginia.

To compute the effects of an increased tax rate requires knowledge of the tax base. As an example, the current rate of taxation in Michigan is 12.5 mills per cigarette, or $0.25 per package of 20 cigarettes. At this rate the tax generates $268 million (FY89 DMB estimate) in revenue. The tax base is therefore 1.072 billion packages of cigarettes. A contemplated tax increase of $.05 would then be expected to raise approximately $53.6 million in revenue. This, of course, assumes present rates of consumption will hold constant, which is not a realistic assumption.

Research on smoking indicates that the price elasticity of demand is about −0.35, indicating that a 10 percent change in price would lead to a 3.5 percent reduction in the quantity of cigarettes demanded. This relatively weak price response reflects the addictive nature of cigarettes and suggests that efforts to reduce smoking by raising the price of cigarettes (within politically acceptable limits) through higher taxes may be ineffective. It also indicates that an increased tax on cigarettes would lead to some reduction in the quantity demanded and therefore less tax revenue than might first be expected. In addition, with smoking habits on the decline, the tax base may be diminishing over time.

Continuing the example of a $.05 increase, we would expect that tax increase to reduce consumption of cigarettes by about 1.4 percent (.35 times .05), making the new tax base 1.057 billion packages of cigarettes. Hence, the tax will raise $52.8 million in revenue, not $53.6 million as first supposed.

This elasticity estimate is also useful in assessing the extent to which the tax increase will reduce smoking and thus improve health. It is often argued that a tax increase on cigarettes will be beneficial due to its effect of discouraging smoking. As the above estimates indicate, the impact of the tax increase is modest, however. Any substantial reduction in smoking would require very large increases in taxation. Taxation

Table 2
State Cigarette Tax Rates Per Package, 1989
(local taxes not included)

New England		Southeast	
Connecticut	.40	Alabama	.165
Maine	.31	Arkansas	.21
Massachusetts	.26	Florida	.24
New Hampshire	.21	Georgia	.12
Rhode Island	.37	Kentucky	.03
Vermont	.17	Louisiana	.16
		Mississippi	.18
Mideast		North Carolina	.02
Delaware	.14	South Carolina	.07
D.C.	.17	Tennessee	.13
Maryland	.13	Virginia	.025
New Jersey	.27	West Virginia	.17
New York	.33		
Pennsylvania	.18	Southwest	
		Arizona	.15
Great Lakes		New Mexico	.15
Illinois	.30	Oklahoma	.23
Indiana	.155	Texas	.26
Michigan	.25		
Ohio	.18	Rocky Mountain	
Wisconsin	.30	Colorado	.20
		Idaho	.18
Plains		Montana	.18
Iowa	.31	Utah	.23
Kansas	.24	Wyoming	.12
Minnesota	.38		
Missouri	.13	Far West	
Nebraska	.27	California	.35
North Dakota	.30	Nevada	.30
South Dakota	.23	Oregon	.28
		Washington	.34
		Alaska	.29
		Hawaii	40 percent of wholesale price

SOURCES: ACIR's *Significant Features of Fiscal Federalism,* 1989 Edition, Volume 1; and Tobacco Institute of America data.

is simply a very ineffective method of reducing smoking. That is not to say, however, that a tax increase will not be more or less important in affecting the smoking behavior of a given group of people in society. It has been suggested that young smokers, just getting started in the habit, may be more responsive to prices than older smokers. If that is the case, a tax increase may be somewhat more effective for that group.

Recent studies, such as Manning et al. (1989), also suggest that the present level of cigarette taxation, both state and federal, in the United States is at the correct level to compensate for the social costs imposed by smoking. This result, together with potential border problems associated with differential state cigarette tax rates, suggests that other revenue sources be investigated for improved health care access.

The cigarette tax should be levied in an *ad valorem* manner, perhaps as a percentage of the wholesale price of the product, in order to avoid the problem that a unit tax generates less real revenue over time as inflation erodes the value of the tax. A unit tax must be adjusted periodically to maintain its real revenue-generating ability. This process is time-consuming and politically troublesome as the question of the level of taxation is re-examined. Currently, Hawaii is the only state to levy a cigarette tax in an *ad valorem* manner. Their tax is 40 percent of the wholesale price per package of cigarettes.

Alcoholic Beverage Tax Rate Change

Taxation of alcoholic beverages typically includes excise taxes on beer, wine, and liquor. A specific tax is sometimes also applied to liquor. Rates of taxation on these commodities can be adjusted to generate more revenue and also help pay the costs associated with externalities caused by their consumption. Recent studies of the social costs associated with the consumption of alcoholic beverages suggests that present levels of federal and state taxation only cover about half of the external costs. As a result, a substantial increase in taxation may be justified at either the federal or state (or both) levels. See Pogue and Sgontz (1989) and Manning et al. (1989) on this issue.

Estimates of the price and income elasticities of demand for alcoholic beverages are presented in Table 3 (Marshall 1985). The own-price elasticities of demand are small for both beer and wine (–0.76 and –0.50 respectively) indicating that the quantity demanded is not very sensitive to changes in the good's own price. A 10 percent increase in its price would lead to a 7.6 percent reduction in the quantity of beer demanded, and for wine, a 5 percent reduction in the quantity demanded. The price elasticity of demand for spirits is unitary, indicating that a given percentage change in price will lead to a proportionate percentage change in the quantity demanded.

Table 3
Alcoholic Beverage Elasticities

Beverage	Beer price	Wine price	Spirits price	Income
Beer	–0.76	0.12	0.63	0.23
Wine	0.09	–0.50	0.31	2.00
Spirits	0.61	0.33	–1.00	1.27

SOURCE: Marshall (1985).

There are several implications that follow from these elasticity estimates. First, since the demand for beer and wine is inelastic, tax increases on these commodities will result in higher revenues. As the price rises due to a tax increase, the quantity demanded falls, but not proportionately. Consequently, tax revenues rise with tax rate increases. A second implication of the elasticity estimates for alcoholic beverages is that a tax increase on beer or wine will be borne by the consumer to a greater extent than an increase in the tax on spirits. With relatively inelastic demand, the consumer bears a greater share of the tax burden than the producer (for a given elasticity of supply). The final implication is that the cross-price elasticities indicate the strength of substitutability among the alcoholic beverages. Note that beer and wine are not close substitutes, since their cross-price elasticities are nearly zero. The cross-price elasticities are greater for spirits and beer, but are still less than unitary. In general, the cross-price elasticities indicate that the three forms of alcoholic beverages are not very close substitutes.

As a result, an increased tax on one form of alcoholic beverage will not affect the quantity of other beverages demanded to a significant degree.

The income elasticity estimates indicate that beer consumption does not rise proportionately with increased income, while wine and spirits rise more than proportionately with income. Increased taxes on beer will be regressive, while increased taxes on wine and spirits will be progressive.[10]

Border crossing due to alcoholic beverage tax rate differentials may be a problem, as with cigarette tax differentials. The problem is expected to be smaller in the case of beer, wine, and liquor taxes, however, due to the higher cost of transporting the goods.

Many states are currently proposing increased taxes on alcoholic beverages, however. The Distilled Spirits Council reports that 30 states have proposed tax increases in 1989, while 7 have actually adopted increases, 2 states having increased their taxes by 50 percent.[11] If neighboring states were also to increase their taxes on alcoholic beverages, the potential border problems would be lessened.

Taxation of alcoholic beverages cannot be analyzed in the absence of information on the state distribution methods as well. States either have a controlled distribution system (monopoly distribution) or an open method of distribution (relying on licensing of distributors). The taxation of alcoholic beverages is closely tied with the pricing of the beverages, which is directly tied to the distribution method. While a full discussion of the issues involved is beyond the scope of this chapter, it must be stressed that both sets of issues should be considered. See Fisher (1988) for a good discussion of the issues involved.

Income and Payroll Tax Sources

Payroll Tax

A natural way to pay for health care access is through a payroll tax mechanism. Wages and salaries would be subject to a tax of a given percentage, perhaps shared equally by employer and employee. The tax would apply to personal earnings only. Capital income is not taxed under the payroll tax. The social security tax is a good example of this type of tax; employer and employee both pay 7.65 percent, up to a maximum taxable wage of $51,300. The precise tax rate needed would depend upon the tax base and the revenue needs of the access improvement program. A payroll tax is simple to administer and capable of generating large amounts of revenue.

As an example of the potential application of payroll taxes to fund health care access, consider Ohio House Bill 425, introduced during the 1989-90 regular session of the General Assembly. That bill establishes a universal health insurance plan funded through a payroll tax of 8 percent to be paid by employers together with a 1 percent wage tax and a 2 percent tax on interest and dividends to be paid by individuals. In this case, the distribution of tax burden is affected by the combination of taxes and differing rates.

Of course, the incidence of a payroll tax is not what it appears. If we first consider personal earnings, it is clear that the specification of a cap, beyond which the marginal tax rate is zero, means that the tax is proportional up to the cap and regressive thereafter. Taking a broader view of income, and including capital income (interest and dividends), makes the payroll tax even more regressive overall. Musgrave and Musgrave (1989) note that the payroll tax is largely a regressive tax since the share of capital earnings rises with income. Further, while employer and employee appear to share the tax burden equally, the employer is able to shift part of the tax to the employee through lower wages than would be paid in the absence of the tax.

As an example of a payroll tax approach to fund improved health care access, consider such a tax on uninsured workers to provide access. Simulating such a tax for the State of Michigan, Goddeeris finds, in chapter 4 of this volume, that a tax of 10 percent on wages and salaries for adult workers not covered by group insurance in their own names would generate $430 million in revenue.

Income Tax Rate Change

Forty of the states have comprehensive income taxes with marginal tax rates ranging from about 1 percent to 12 percent.[12] Five of these states have flat rate taxes, while the remainder have progressive rate structures.[13] One method of raising revenue is to raise tax rates. To estimate potential revenues, one must know the tax base—the state definition of taxable income—and apply the increase in rate to it to compute new revenues that would be generated. State income tax structures are often complex, and detailed knowledge of the specific provisions of tax law are required. As an example, Michigan's flat rate income tax is applied at the rate of 4.6 percent to taxable income based on the federal definition of adjusted gross income. The tax generates $3.6 billion (FY 1989 estimate). Taking the broadest possible definition of the tax base (no effective exemptions, no credits, no deductions), an additional 1 percent tax will generate nearly $1 billion in revenue. Other state income tax structures can be analyzed similarly to determine the revenue response likely from a given change in tax rate. It should be noted that such rough rules of thumb ignore elasticity responses. Higher income tax rates will alter the level of economic activity in the state and ultimately affect the tax base.

Income Tax Base Changes

Twenty-three of the 40 states with comprehensive income taxes use federal adjusted gross income (AGI) as the starting point in defining taxable income.[14] As a consequence, federal tax preferences generally apply at the state level as well. For example, the favorable tax treatment of benefits compared to wages applies to state tax structures as well. Since benefits are not included in the definition of AGI, they are generally not taxed at the state level either. As a result, the tax system distorts the choice between wage/salary income and benefits. Another large tax preference is provided for owner-occupied housing, because the value of housing services provided by a home is tax-exempt. Other capital assets generating income are taxed.

Other examples could be cited but these two are sufficient to make the point that the current definition of income is rather narrow.[15] Taxing some of these forms of income would generate additional revenues for health care access.

Economists have suggested several base-broadening measures for the federal income tax which may also be relevant for state income taxes.

Table 4 provides Joseph Pechman's estimates of the broadening in taxable income which would follow from less liberal personal deductions, taxing some transfer payments, taxing fringe benefits, and alteration of the two-earner deduction. These base-broadening measures would increase federal taxable income by 15.7 percent, compared to the 1986 definition. The amount by which a state's tax revenue would rise depends upon several factors, including: (a) the nature of the state's tax base and the link between the state's tax code and the federal code (i.e., whether the state has adopted the federal definition of AGI for taxable income); and (b) the state's marginal tax rate structure. State-specific estimates of the revenue implications of base-broadening measures require this information, together with assumptions regarding the behavioral changes likely to be prompted by the change in tax base.

Table 4
Alternative Personal Income Tax Base
(billions of dollars)

Item	Adjusted gross income (AGI)	Taxable income
Tax Reform Act of 1986	$3,545	$2,407
Plus:		
Personal deductions	0	68
Transfer payments	226	164
Fringe benefits	187	185
Two-earner deduction	-82	-81
Other	43	42
Equals: comprehensive tax	$3,919	$2,785

SOURCE: Congressional Budget Office, as reported in Pechman (1987).

Tax Benefits

The suggestion to tax fringe benefits alone would generate an additional $37 billion in federal revenue, assuming an average marginal tax rate of 20 percent. More specifically, consider the taxation of health insurance premiums provided by employers. The rationale for this approach lies in the observation that the present income tax base includes wage and salary income but not benefits provided by the employer. An additional dollar of salary is taxed at a 15 percent, 28 percent or 33 percent rate by the federal government, plus a state tax rate of perhaps 5 percent, while additional benefits are not taxed at all. As a result, there is a clear incentive for employees to request benefits in place of some money income.[16] From an individual's point of view, the choice is clear. If a person would have purchased a $1,200 health insurance policy anyway, receiving the benefit of the policy rather than $1,200 in salary saves the typical taxpayer $336 in federal income taxes (assuming the individual is in the 28 percent tax bracket). To remove this distortion from the tax system, and to take away the substantial subsidy involved, the insurance premium paid by the employer on behalf of the employee could be counted as taxable income.

States can consider several variants of this proposal: (a) taxing the first x dollars of coverage; (b) taxing all coverage provided; or (c) taxing coverage over x dollars. The first approach was included in the 1981 proposal for federal tax reform, which contained a provision taxing the first $10 per month ($120 per year) for a single filer or $25 per month ($300 per year) for a married filer. As an example of the state level impact, that proposal would have increased the Michigan income tax liability of Michigan residents by $24 million. In addition to the revenue impact of the proposal, a state needs to consider the distributional consequences. Simulations performed by the Michigan Department of Treasury indicated that this proposal would have reduced tax liability for 20,688 Michigan income tax filers by a total of $51,000 while increasing tax liability for 2,309,740 filers, raising their taxes by $24.305 million.[17] Most of the impact of this proposal would have been felt by taxpayers with adjusted gross income in the $30,000 to $50,000 range. In fact, 60 percent of the total tax increase is borne by taxpayers with AGI of $30,000 or more. Low-income taxpayers, with AGI less than $15,000, would bear 12 percent of the tax burden.

Such a proposal is misdirected, however, being very regressive in only taxing the first $120 or $300 of benefits. Above these levels, the marginal tax rate would be zero. From a state tax policy perspective, it would be better for a state to exempt the first x dollars of benefits and to tax benefits above that level. In this way, the tax would be somewhat progressive and treat wages and benefits equally, above some basic level of benefits.

The exclusion of health care benefits from taxation results in substantial loss of revenue. Pechman (1987) reports that the tax expenditure associated with the exclusion of employer contributions to medical insurance premiums and medical care at the federal level is $30.205 billion (1988 estimate). Additional revenues are involved at the state level as well. For example, the Michigan Department of Treasury estimates that taxing all employer contributions to health and life insurance would generate $296 million in state income tax revenue.[18] Removing the life insurance portion of this total may reduce the current tax expenditure to $250 million. For equity and efficiency reasons, however, there is no reason to separate the two types of insurance—both should be taxed.

Tax Lottery Winnings

States with lotteries can consider broadening the income tax base to include lottery winnings, if they are not currently taxed. Lottery winnings are taxable at the federal level, but not at the state level in all states with lotteries. At the federal level, gamblers are permitted to deduct losses, paying tax on net winnings, which cannot be done on some state income taxes. As an example of the revenue potential here, consider the Michigan case where taxation of lottery winnings is estimated to generate $24 million in revenue.

The incidence of the lottery tax has been investigated by Suits (1982). He found that the lottery is twice as regressive as the second most regressive tax—the sales tax. From this perspective, additional reliance on a very regressive tax is not a just change in tax policy. Arguments that the regressivity of the lottery does not matter because it is a voluntary tax are specious.

Tax Employer Contributions to Pensions or Social Security

The exclusion of net pension contributions and earnings results in a sizable amount of lost tax revenue. Pechman (1987) reports that the exclusion of employer plans results in a tax expenditure of $58.185

billion at the federal level, while the exclusion of IRA contributions results in a loss of $11.635 billion, and Keogh plans add another $1.715 billion. The exclusion of social security income also results in a substantial revenue loss. Taxing OASI benefits for retired workers would generate an additional $12.025 billion in federal revenue, while taxing benefits for dependents and survivors would generate $3.545 billion, and disability insurance benefits would generate $1.040 billion. State revenues involved are less, of course, depending upon state tax base definition and marginal tax rates.

Taxing employer contributions to pension plans or taxing social security income would generate large revenues for states, but both of these tax expenditures have strong political support and are unlikely targets for added revenue. States can at least conform to the federal definition of taxable income in this regard. For example, a state could at least tax that portion of social security income which the federal government taxes. In Michigan, for example, this would generate an additional $27.5 million in revenue.[19]

A recent Supreme Court ruling requires that states tax state and federal pension income alike, rather than exempting state pension income and taxing federal pension income as some states currently do.

Business Taxation

Table 5 illustrates the many ways in which states have chosen to tax business activity. While all states tax business activity, and a number tax it several different ways, there is a wide variety of tax mechanisms employed. Most states rely on a corporate income tax for about 4 to 5 percent of state general revenue. Some states use gross receipts taxes (Hawaii, Indiana, West Virginia, and Washington) and one state uses a value-added tax (Michigan). Forty-nine of the states also have corporate license taxes, and all 50 tax insurance premiums. In addition, 33 states levy severance taxes on natural resources.

Since states use very diverse methods of taxing business activity, it is difficult to generalize about potential revenues. Revenues can certainly be raised by increasing the rate of taxation, whether it be based on corporate profits, gross receipts, or value-added. Aside from rate change, though, most states' business tax structures are replete with myriad forms of business tax expenditures. Consideration should be given to repeal of specific exemptions which may no longer be effective in accomplishing the stated objective. Tax preferences for specific industries, or for specific firms for that matter, may not serve legitimate state policy objectives and may be targeted for potential revenue. Analysis of the incidence of the state business tax structure is a necessary prerequisite for making such changes. After determining that specific industries pay more or less than their share of state business taxes, tax policy changes can be recommended.

Table 5
State Business Taxes

Type of tax	Number of states	Tax revenue ($ billion, 1985)	Percent of state general revenue
Corporate income tax	45	16.915	4.3
Gross receipts tax	4	1.670	0.4
Value-added tax	1	1.448	0.4
Corporate license tax	49	3.065	0.8
Severance tax	33	6.125	1.6
Insurance premiums tax	50	5.489	1.4

SOURCE: Fisher (1988), p. 215.

Transition From Business Provision
of Health Insurance to State Insurance Plan

An important policy suggestion which states are grappling with centers on the question: Who pays for health insurance? The tradition, coming from years of collective bargaining and cultural expectations, has been that the employer provides health insurance and other benefits. This is quite reasonable, especially in light of the tax incentives involved. Employees can receive insurance at substantially subsidized rates by having the employer pay the premium, which is exempt from federal and state income taxation. Recent pressures for U.S. industry to become more competitive in world markets, however, force firms to reconsider the provision of such benefits. A specific proposal to move from employer-provided health benefits to a more universal health care system, provided by the states, has been suggested (see chapter 3). Of course, the major economic stumbling block in this proposal lies in the fact that the health insurance benefits become taxable when moved out of the workplace under current tax law. With changes in tax law, creative solutions to the transition may be forthcoming. In the absence of such changes, the penalty for such a change is severe.

Issues of Federalism

Deductibility Issues

Federal deductibility of state taxes has several important implications for state tax systems.[20] First, with federal deductibility states may have more progressive tax structures than they would otherwise. The high-income taxpayers, who pay the higher marginal tax rates at the state level, are also more likely to itemize on their federal returns, deducting the state taxes and lowering their federal tax liability. A second implication of deductibility is that states can collect more revenue than they could in the absence of deductibility. Deductibility can induce some taxpayers to support higher state taxes than they otherwise would since it reduces the net marginal tax price of an added dollar of increased state expenditure. Finally, deductibility dampens interstate tax differences. If taxes are $300 higher for a given individual in State A compared to State B, the deductibility of state taxes reduces that difference to $216 (assuming the taxpayer is in the 28 percent marginal tax bracket and there is no deductibility at the state level).

Understanding these deductibility implications has relevance to the choice of a tax instrument for financing improved health care access. Choosing a deductible tax, such as the income tax, brings with it all of these implications. Choosing a nondeductible tax, such as the sales tax, does not. While there are certainly other issues to consider, these implications must be part of the policy discussion in selecting a tax-based financing method.

Since the Tax Reform Act of 1986, state (and local) sales taxes are no longer deductible from federal adjusted gross income. As a result, increases in the sales tax rate would cost itemizing taxpayers an additional 15 percent, 28 percent, or 33 percent, depending on their tax bracket, when compared to financing that relies on a deductible tax. Nonitemizers, of course, would not be affected by the nondeductibility of the sales tax. As an example of a typical case, consider a state where 35 percent of federal income tax returns filed by taxpayers included itemization. If the average marginal tax rate for those taxpayers is 20 percent, then an additional dollar of revenue raised in the state through a nondeductible sales tax would cost the taxpayers $1.00 compared to $0.93 if the same revenue were raised using a deductible tax. The 7 percent difference is the premium a state pays if it chooses to fund health care access using the nondeductible tax. The federal government has given states the clear incentive to finance new activity with income or property taxes, not sales taxes.

Tax/Revenue Limitations

A number of states have enacted revenue or expenditure limitations since California led the way with Proposition 13 in 1978. Notable among the state limitations are Massachusetts' Proposition 2-1/2, which is a property tax limitation, and Michigan's Headlee Amendment, which limits all state revenues. With such limitations in place, states must consider the implications of new funding mechanisms proposed to improve health care access. For example, a new tax source that would generate several hundred million dollars in revenue in Michigan would violate the Headlee Amendment, requiring either dramatic reductions in other taxes or a change in the state constitution, neither of which is attractive.

Summary and Conclusions

A number of potential revenue sources for financing improved access to health care have been identified in this chapter. The choice of which funding mechanism is best for a given policy proposal is complex. For access proposals that are relatively cheap ($100 million), some combination of increased taxes on alcoholic beverages, prescription drugs, or amusement services can be used. More comprehensive policy proposals carrying higher price tags ($400 to $600 million) will require correspondingly more substantial tax policy changes. Including some services in the sales tax base (perhaps coupled with a sales tax credit on the income tax to relieve regressivity), taxing employer contributions to health and life insurance under the state income tax, or levying a payroll tax are all possibilities. For any given policy proposal, the appropriate funding mechanism should be identified not only on the basis of the revenue generated, but also with regard to the incidence and incentive effects of the mechanism.

NOTES

1. The notion of a tax expenditure comes from a budgeting perspective that acknowledges that when a tax system exempts certain activity from taxation, the preferential treatment is equivalent to a direct budget expenditure for that activity. Hence, the amount of the tax exemption or preferential treatment is termed a tax expenditure.

2. ACIR (1991).

3. A use tax is a form of sales tax due on goods used but not purchased in the state. For example, a sales tax is levied on a pair of shoes purchased in the state, but a use tax is levied on a pair purchased from a mail order firm in another state. As another example, a sales tax is applied to the purchase of a new car, a use tax is applied to the lease of a new car. The use tax is designed to close common sales tax loopholes.

4. State of Michigan Executive Budget, Tax Expenditure Appendix, 1987-88 Fiscal Year, p. 39.

5. For a discussion of the economic issues involved, see Fox and Murray (1988).

6. It should be noted that recent research using computational general equilibrium methods finds that taxing services under the sales tax may be less regressive than traditional theory suggests. The reason is due to the reduction (increase) in labor supply by lower- (higher-) income households. For the low-income households, the income effect of a higher cost-of-living due to the sales tax on services appears to dominate the income effect of wages, resulting in upward sloping labor supply curves with respect to both wages and the cost-of-living. For further discussion of this view, see Baum (1991).

7. It must be noted that transportation costs are a factor to consider as well.

8. See ACIR (1986).

9. This section discusses taxation of cigarettes, but other forms of tobacco should be taxed in similar ways. That would include cigars, pipe tobacco, and chewing tobacco products. To avoid distortions in the system, all tobacco products should be taxed at the same rate.

10. Some caution is needed in making this generalization, since the elasticity estimates are point estimates—evaluated at a mean level of income—and do not hold precisely over the income distribution.

11. *Wall Street Journal*, July 12, 1989.

12. Those states with no income tax are: Alaska, Florida, Nevada, South Dakota, Texas, Washington, and Wyoming. States with limited income taxes are: Connecticut, New Hampshire, and Tennessee.

13. Those with flat rate taxes are: Massachusetts, Pennsylvania, Illinois, Indiana, and Michigan (ACIR 1989).

14. ACIR (1988; 1989).

15. See Pechman (1987).

16. See Woodbury (1989).

17. Michigan Department of Treasury (1986).

18. Michigan Department of Management and Budget (1987-88).

19. Federal income tax liability occurs when half of the social security benefits plus modified adjusted gross income is more than $32,000 on a joint return ($25,000 on a single return). The federal tax applies to half of the excess, or half of the social security income, whichever is less. Michigan does not tax this income.

20. The reasons cited here are adapted from Fisher (1988).

References

Advisory Commission on Intergovernmental Relations (ACIR). 1986. *State and Local Taxation of Out-of-State Mail Order Sales,* Report A-105, Washington, DC.

_____. 1989. *Significant Features of Fiscal Federalism,* Volume 1, Washington, DC.

Baum, Donald N. 1991. "Economic Effects of Including Services in the Sales Tax Base: An Applied General Equilibrium Analysis," *Public Finance Quarterly* 19(2): 166-92.

Blair, Andrew R., Frank Giarratani, and Michael H. Spiro. 1987. "Incidence of the Amusement Tax," *National Tax Journal* 60(1): 61-69.

Bohm, Robert A. and Eleanor D. Craig. 1987. "Sales Tax Base Modification, Revenue Stability and Equity," National Tax Association-Tax Institute of America, *Proceedings of the Eightieth Annual Conference,* pp. 167-74.

Fisher, Ronald C. 1988. *State and Local Public Finance.* Glenview, IL: Scott Foresman.

Fox, William F. and Matthew Murray. 1988. "Economic Aspects of Taxing Services," *National Tax Journal* 61(1): 19-36.

Hellerstein, Walter. 1988. "Florida's Sales Tax on Services," *National Tax Journal* 61(1): 1-18.

Manning, Willard G., Emmett B. Keeler, Joseph P. Newhouse, Elizabeth M. Sloss, and Jeffrey Wasserman. 1989. "The Taxes of Sin: Do Smokers and Drinkers Pay Their Way?" *JAMA* 261(11): 1604-1609.

Marshall, Gary L. 1985. "Developing a State Alcohol Beverage Simulation Model," National Tax Association-Tax Institute of America, *Proceedings of the Seventy-Eighth Annual Conference,* pp. 180-86.

Michigan Department of Management and Budget. 1987-88. *State of Michigan Executive Budget, Tax Expenditure Appendix.* Lansing, MI.

Michigan Department of Treasury, Taxation and Economic Policy Office. 1986. "The Impacts of Federal Tax Reform in Michigan: Analysis of House and Senate Plans." Lansing, MI.

_____. 1985. "Analysis of the Michigan Single Business Tax." Lansing, MI.

Musgrave, Richard A. and Peggy B. Musgrave. 1989. *Public Finance In Theory and Practice.* NY: McGraw-Hill.

Ohio House Bill #425, 118th General Assembly Regular Session, 1989-90.

Pechman, Joseph A. 1990. "The Future of the Income Tax." *American Economic Review* 80(1): 1-20.

_____. 1987. *Federal Tax Policy,* 5th ed. Washington, DC: The Brookings Institution.

Pogue, Thomas F. and Larry G. Sgontz. 1989. "Taxing to Control Social Costs: The Case of Alcohol," *American Economic Review* 79(1): 235-43.

Suits, Daniel B. 1982. "Gambling as a Source of Revenue." In *Michigan's Fiscal and Economic Structure,* eds. Harvey E. Brazer and Deborah S. Laren. Ann Arbor: University of Michigan Press.

Woodbury, Stephen A. 1989. "The Use of Tax Reduction or Subsidies to Encourage Coverage of the Employed Uninsured—Supplement to Preliminary Report to the Governor's Task Force on Access to Health Care." Lansing, MI.

8
Labor Market Impacts of Policies to Expand Access to Health Care

Stephen A, Woodbury
Andrew J. Hogan
Michigan State University

In the United States, private health insurance coverage is closely tied to employment—most individuals who are covered by private health insurance receive it either as part of their compensation for employment or through a family member who receives it as part of his or her compensation. As a result, policies designed to alter health care provision may have the side effect of influencing labor markets. That is, policy-induced changes in the health care system can be expected to alter the mix of employment, total employment, and wages.

This paper examines how various policies intended to expand health insurance coverage in a state may also affect that state's labor market. The first section of the paper provides background data on the U.S. labor market; it explores the relationships among hourly wages, inclusion in an employer-provided group health plan, and coverage by any form of health insurance. Also provided are data on wages and health insurance coverage by industry. The second section of the paper develops the linkages between changes in health care policy and changes in wages and employment. Although we offer predictions about the qualitative impact of the policies (that is, directions of the policies' impacts on the labor market), we are reluctant to make precise quantitative predictions because little of the empirical work needed to offer quantitative estimates of wage and employment impacts has been performed.

The Labor Market and Health Insurance

Table 1 shows the distribution of hourly wage and salary earnings in the United States in 1988 (see the first two columns). The figures show that nearly 2.7 million workers earned less than the minimum wage of $3.35 in 1988, and that another 6.8 million earned from $3.35 to $4.00 an hour. (Hourly earnings below the minimum wage are possible because of incomplete coverage of the Fair Labor Standards Act and because of imperfect compliance with the Act.) It follows that nearly 9.5 million workers—or about 11 percent of all wage and salary workers in the United States—had earnings near or below the minimum wage in 1988.

Table 1 also shows that an additional 8.3 million workers had hourly earnings of $4.01 to $5.00 in 1988. If we characterize all workers with earnings at or below $5.00 per hour as *low-wage*, then a total of 17.8 million workers in 1988—or over 20 percent of all wage and salary workers in the United States—would be characterized as low-wage.

Table 1 also shows that the inclusion of workers in employer-provided group health insurance plans is strongly correlated with hourly earnings (see the columns headed "Included in Group Health Plan"). Workers whose hourly earnings were $5.00 or less were far less likely to be included in an employer-provided health insurance plan than were workers whose hourly earnings were above $5.00. Only about 13 percent of workers with hourly earnings below $3.35 were included in an employer-provided health insurance plan, whereas nearly 88 percent of workers with hourly earnings over $15.00 were included.

Finally, Table 1 shows that even though low-wage workers are far less likely than high-wage workers to be included in employer-provided health insurance plans, they are only slightly less likely than high-wage workers to be covered by *any* form of health insurance (see columns headed "Covered by Any Health Insurance"). Low-wage workers—those earning $5.00 or less per hour—had roughly an 80 percent probability of being covered by any form of health insurance, whereas workers earning over $5.00 per hour had better than a 90 percent probability of being covered. The difference between the percentages of

Table 1

Inclusion of U.S. Workers in Group Health Plans,
by Hourly Wage and Salary Earnings, 1988

Hourly wage and salary earnings	Total number of workers (1,000s)	Included in group health plan		Covered by any health insurance	
		Number of workers (1,000s)	Percent of total	Number of workers (1,000s)	Percent of total
Less than $3.35	2,674	346	12.9	2,068	77.3
$3.35 – $4.00	6,816	1,282	18.8	5,329	78.2
$4.01 – $5.00	8,267	3,097	37.5	7,107	86.0
$5.01 – $7.50	19,150	11,487	60.0	17,600	91.9
$7.51 – $10.00	17,203	12,936	75.2	16,507	95.9
$10.01 – $15.00	19,849	16,755	84.4	19,508	98.3
Over $15.01	13,613	11,962	87.8	13,502	99.0
All workers	87,590	57,865	66.1	81,621	93.2

NOTES: Figures displayed are authors' tabulations from the May 1988 Current Population Survey. The sample includes wage and salary workers who responded to the May Employee Benefits Supplement and reported information about occupation and industry of employment. Military and self-employed workers are excluded.

low-wage and high-wage workers who are covered by any health insurance is far less than the difference between the percentages of low-
wage and high-wage workers who are included in an employer-provided
group health plan. The reason is that most low-wage workers are either
covered by a public program or are part of a family in which someone
else's health insurance extends to the low-wage workers.

Table 1 suggests the importance of designing health care access policies
that target the uninsured. In particular, the figures suggest that policies
designed to include more workers as the primary insured in employer-
provided health plans are less likely to target uninsured individuals than
are policies that act directly to cover uninsured individuals. The reason
is simply that most individuals who work in the labor market are,
regardless of their hourly earnings, covered by some form of health
insurance. Including more workers as the primary insured in employer-
provided group health plans would result in the addition (as primary
insureds) of many workers who are already covered by some form of
health insurance.

In Table 2, the same sample of workers is broken down by industry
of employment. The first two columns show that by far the largest sectors of the economy are professional and related services, retail trade,
and durable goods manufacturing. The column labeled "Included in
Group Health Plan" shows that there is much interindustry variation
in the percentage of workers who are included in employer-provided
health plans. In several industries, more than 70 percent of all workers
were included in employer-provided group health plans: mining, durable
and nondurable goods manufacturing, transportation, wholesale trade,
finance, and public administration. But in other industries—agriculture,
retail trade, and personal services—only about 30 to 40 percent of all
workers were included. It follows that policies to expand the inclusion
of workers in employer-provided health plans would probably have an
uneven impact, affecting mainly industries in which health insurance
provision tends to be low.

Although there is much industry-to-industry variation in the percentage of workers included in employer-provided health plans, Table 2
also shows that there is far less industry-to-industry variation in the
percentage of workers who are covered by any health insurance (see

Table 2
Inclusion of U.S. Wage and Salary Workers
in Group Health Plans by Industry of Employment, 1988

Industry	Total number of workers (1,000s)	Included in group health plan		Covered by any health insurance	
		Number of workers (1,000s)	Percent of total	Number of workers (1,000s)	Percent of total
Agriculture, forestry, fisheries	1,468	443	30.2	1,060	72.2
Mining	665	570	85.7	651	97.8
Construction	4,806	2,748	57.2	4,079	84.9
Durable goods	10,578	9,053	85.6	10,287	97.2
Nondurable goods	7,982	6,299	78.9	7,636	95.7
Transportation, communications, public utilities	6,382	5,342	83.7	6,139	96.2
Wholesale trade	3,490	2,568	73.6	3,348	95.9
Retail trade	14,211	6,095	42.9	12,506	88.0
Finance, insurance, real estate	6,415	4,658	72.6	6,165	96.1
Business and repair services	4,072	2,198	54.0	3,588	88.1
Personal services	2,540	813	32.0	2,153	84.8
Entertainment and recreation services	894	415	46.3	775	86.6
Professional and related services	19,267	12,651	65.7	18,503	96.0
Public administration	4,820	4,014	83.3	4,732	98.2
All workers	87,590	57,865	66.1	81,621	93.2

NOTES: Figures displayed are authors' tabulations from the May 1988 Current Population Survey. The sample includes wage and salary workers who responded to the May Employee Benefits Supplement and reported information about occupation and industry of employment. Military and self-employed workers are excluded.

columns labeled "Covered by Any Health Insurance"). Only in agriculture is the percentage of workers covered by any health insurance less than 80 percent, and in the four largest industries, the percentage of workers covered is 88 percent or greater. Again, it appears that most workers who are not included in an employer-provided health plan are covered nevertheless by some form of health insurance.

Table 3 shows the distribution of wages within each of the major industries in the United States in 1988. The table shows both the number and percentage of workers in each industry whose hourly wage and salary earnings were under $5.01, from $5.01 to $10.00, and over $10.00. In three industries—agriculture, personal services, and retail trade—at least 45 percent of all workers had hourly wage and salary earnings under $5.01 in 1988. At the high end of the wage scale were mining, durable goods manufacturing, transportation, and public administration. In all of these industries, at least half of all workers had hourly earnings over $10.00 in 1988.

Together, Tables 2 and 3 show that industries that tend to pay high wages also tend to include a high proportion of their workers in employer-provided group health plans. This apparent link between wages and employer-provision of health insurance suggests that high-productivity workers are highly compensated with both wage and non-wage benefits. This link bears implications for how changes in health care policy will affect different industries and groups of workers.

Labor Market Analysis of the Policies

Conventional labor market analysis can provide insights into how various policies to expand health insurance coverage might influence wages and employment. The strategy here is as follows. First, we set out a general labor market model that can be used to analyze the impact of various policies on the labor market outcomes that are of greatest concern: wages and employment. The model involves specifying two sets of factors: those influencing the quantity of labor that workers are willing to supply to a given labor market, and those influencing the quantity of labor that employers will demand from that same labor market.

Table 3
Distribution of U.S. Hourly Wage and Salary Earnings by Industry of Employment, 1988

Industry	Total number of workers (1,000s)	Number (1,000s) and percentage of workers with hourly wage and salary earnings of:					
		Under $5.01		$5.01 – $10.00		Over $10.00	
		Number	Percent	Number	Percent	Number	Percent
Agriculture, forestry, fisheries	1,468	839	57.2	496	33.8	133	9.1
Mining	665	46	6.8	169	25.4	451	67.7
Construction	4,806	587	12.2	2,203	45.8	2,016	41.9
Durable goods	10,578	784	7.4	4,173	39.4	5,621	53.1
Nondurable goods	7,982	1,370	17.2	3,403	42.6	3,209	40.2
Transportation, communications, public utilities	6,382	368	5.8	2,035	31.9	3,979	62.4
Wholesale trade	3,490	471	13.5	1,601	45.9	1,418	40.6
Retail trade	14,211	6,392	45.0	5,751	40.5	2,068	14.5
Finance, insurance, real estate	6,415	640	10.0	3,072	47.9	2,704	42.1
Business and repair services	4,072	933	22.9	1,755	43.1	1,384	34.0
Personal services	2,540	1,397	55.0	971	38.2	172	6.8
Entertainment and recreation services	894	323	36.1	373	41.7	198	22.2
Professional and related services	19,267	3,253	16.9	8,443	43.8	7,571	39.3
Public administration	4,820	355	7.4	1,909	39.6	2,556	53.0
All workers	87,590	17,757	20.3	36,353	41.5	33,480	38.2

NOTES: Figures displayed are authors' tabulations from the May 1988 Current Population Survey. The sample includes wage and salary workers who responded to the May Employee Benefits Supplement and reported information about occupation and industry of employment. Military and self-employed workers are excluded.

Next, we define what we mean by a labor market and discuss the application of the model to the various policies that are of interest. Finally, we use the model to analyze in a general qualitative way the implications of the policies for labor markets. We plan in future work to derive quantitative estimates of how large the predicted effects would be.

The Model

In general, both economic theory and a significant body of empirical work suggest that the amount of labor willingly supplied to a given labor market [or labor supply to market i, LS_i] will depend on five influences: (1) hourly wage and salary earnings paid in that labor market [w_i]; (2) taxes paid by workers on their earnings [t]; (3) nonwage characteristics of work in that labor market [n_i], including the safety and desirability of the work, and the provision of health and pension benefits by the employer; (4) the ease or difficulty of gaining entry to the labor market [e_i] due, for example, to educational of licensing requirements; and (5) opportunities (including earnings) available to workers in other pursuits and other labor markets [w_j]. These considerations can be summarized compactly as a labor supply function, which shows the quantity of labor supplied to labor market i as a function of the factors just described:

$$LS_i = LS_i(w_i; t, n_i, e_i, w_j).$$

The relationship between the quantity of labor supplied to labor market i and the wage in that market can be summarized as a labor supply curve (see Figure 1), which shows that as the wage in labor market i increases, more workers are willing to supply labor to this market, other things equal. Changes in the other factors in the labor supply function [t, n_i, e_i, and w_j] can be shown graphically as shifts of the LS_i curve.[1]

The amount of labor that employers demand from labor market i [LD_i] will depend on the following factors: (1) hourly wage and salary earnings paid in that labor market [w_i]; (2) nonwage costs of employing workers from that labor market [c_i], including training costs, costs of complying with safety regulations, and legally required payroll taxes for social security, unemployment insurance, and workers' compensation; (3) prices of other inputs into production [p_j], including capital

Figure 1
Effects of Universal Health Insurance
on Low-Wage Labor Markets

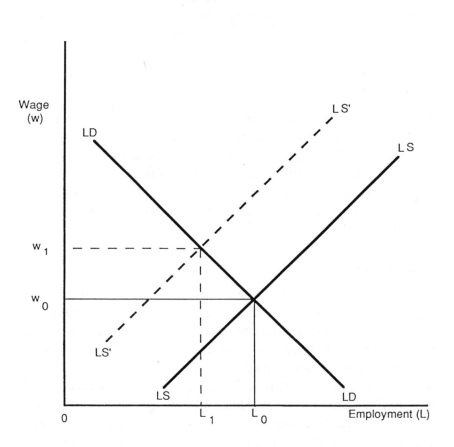

costs and the total cost of employing other kinds of labor; (4) the quantity of output [q] desired by the employer, which may depend in turn on market conditions and current output prices; and (5) the technology of production or organization of the production process [g]. These considerations can be summarized as a labor demand function, which shows the quantity of labor demanded in labor market i as a function of the factors just described:

$$LD_i = LD_i(w_i; c_i, p_j, q, g).$$

The relationship between the quantity of labor demanded from labor market i and the wage in that market can be summarized as a labor demand curve (see Figure 1), which shows that as the wage in labor market i increases, employers will demand less labor from this market, other things equal. Changes in the other factors in the labor demand function [c_i, p_j, q, and g] can be shown graphically as shifts of the LD_i curve.

Applying the Model

The labor market model developed above can be applied to a wide variety of problems. Here we are interested in the labor market impacts of the following policies designed to expand access to health care: (1) universal health insurance managed by the state (chapter 3 in this volume); (2) mandatory employer-provided health insurance, coupled with a public sponsor for those not covered by employer-provided health insurance (chapter 4 in this volume; Mitchell 1989); and (3) a Small Employer Health Insurance Pool, coupled with Medicaid Buy-In programs for the unemployed uninsured and not-in-the-labor-force uninsured (chapters 5.2 and 5.3 in this volume).

We examine the impacts of these policies on two representative labor markets: "low-wage" and "higher-wage." The key assumption we will make about these two labor markets is that *workers in low-wage labor markets do not currently receive employer-provided health insurance* (although they may as a result of policy changes), whereas workers in higher-wage labor markets do. This assumption simplifies the analysis, and is roughly consistent with the empirical findings reported on low- and higher-wage workers.[2]

In addition, it should be understood that low-wage labor markets include a disproportionate number of relatively young workers, minorities, and women, whereas higher-wage labor markets include a disproportionate number of workers aged 25 to 54 who are male. In the labor economics literature, low-wage labor markets are frequently referred to as "low-skill" or "unskilled" labor markets, whereas higher-wage labor markets are referred to as "skilled." These characterizations are intended to be descriptive rather than normative, and there is clearly a whole range of labor markets in between these two types.[3]

Universal Health Insurance

The provision of a specified package of health care services by a single provider to all individuals, regardless of their income or employment status, is universal health insurance. Universal health insurance has become increasingly attractive in recent years because it has the potential both to eliminate incomplete coverage and to bring health care costs under control (chapter 3 in this volume). In view of the possibility that some type of universal plan will be adopted in the future, it is important to understand the labor market effects of such a policy.

Special Assumptions

To analyze the effects of universal health insurance, we adopt the following assumptions. First, we assume that the universal health plan is financed through an increase in personal income tax rates. (If the universal health plan were state-managed, this would imply an increase in state personal income tax rates; if federally managed, it would imply an increase in federal tax rates.)

Second, we assume that the universal health plan will provide health care more efficiently than the current system, in that the total amount of health care provided will increase, but the total resources spent on health care will remain constant. This assumption is one reasonable benchmark, based on the argument that a universal, state-managed, health plan would eliminate administrative and other inefficiencies that are inherent in the current system (see chapter 3 for further discussion).

Third, we assume that workers who are already covered by health insurance will receive health care under a universal plan that is similar to the health care they now receive under their employer-provided plans. The implication of the second and third assumptions is that everyone who is currently covered by health insurance will receive equally good care under the universal plan, and further that individuals who are currently uninsured will receive health care that they would not receive under the current system.

Effects on Low-Wage Labor Markets

The effect of universal health insurance on the supply of low-wage workers is essentially a tax effect. That is, low-wage workers will experience a tax increase that reduces their hourly after-tax earnings. It follows that they will reduce the number of hours they are willing to work at a given before-tax wage (we show this tax effect in Figure 1 by a leftward shift of the labor supply curve from LS to LS').[4]

There would be no effect of the universal plan on the demand for low-wage workers, because we assume that low-wage employers do not currently provide health insurance. As a result, the equilibrium wage in low-wage labor markets would rise, and employment would fall, in response to universal health insurance (see Figure 1). The magnitude of these changes is potentially large, because low-wage workers tend to show a relatively large labor supply response to changes in the real (after-tax) wage.[5]

Effects on Higher-Wage Labor Markets

The effects of universal health insurance on higher-wage labor markets are more complex. Consider first the effect of a universal plan on the supply of higher-wage labor. The tax effect would again apply—higher-wage workers will experience a tax increase that would reduce the number of hours they are willing to work at a given before-tax wage. We would expect this tax effect to be smaller than the tax effect for low-wage workers, because empirical evidence shows that the labor supply of higher-wage workers tends to be relatively insensitive to changes in the real wage. Accordingly, we show the tax effect by a small shift of the supply curve, from LS to LS' in Figure 2.[6]

In addition to the tax effect, there will be a loss-of-benefit effect on the labor supply of high-wage workers. Universal health insurance

Figure 2
Effects of Universal Health Insurance
on Higher-Wage Labor Markets

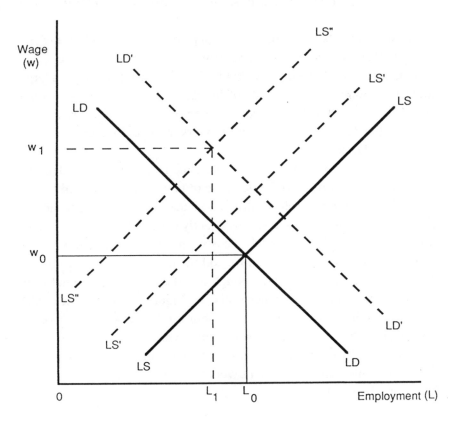

would essentially sever the link between employment and the availability of health insurance. As a result, individuals would no longer need to be employed in order to receive health insurance, and an important non-wage aspect of employment would be eliminated. It follows that labor supply would be further reduced (see the shift from LS' to LS'' in Figure 2).[7]

Consider now the effect of a universal plan on the demand for higher-wage workers. Because higher-wage employers currently provide health insurance, the adoption of universal health insurance could have a large impact on nonwage labor costs of higher-wage employers—it would eliminate the need to pay directly for employees' health insurance. As a result, the demand for higher-wage workers would increase (see the shift from LD to LD' in Figure 2).

Given the assumptions we have made, the increase in labor demand would be in proportion to the decrease in labor supply induced by the loss-of-benefit effect. It follows that, absent the tax effect on labor supply, the equilibrium wage would rise by exactly enough to offset the reduction in employers' nonwage labor costs, and equilibrium employment would be unchanged. But when we add the tax effect, the equilibrium wage increases by more than enough to offset the loss of benefit; as a result, equilibrium employment falls (see Figure 2). Hence, the model does not predict a reduction of total labor costs following adoption of universal health insurance, as some employers appear to expect. On the contrary, the model suggests that total labor costs would rise somewhat, and that employment would fall, in both higher-wage and low-wage labor markets.

Effects if Efficiency Gains Were Small

It is also important to consider how violations of the second and third assumptions made above would change our predictions. That is, what would happen if the efficiency gains from the universal health plan were small, so that even though the total resources devoted to health care would be unchanged, the process of expanding coverage to all individuals reduced average access to health care? In this case, employers would still be relieved of the direct burden of health insurance premiums, and the tax effect on labor supply would still occur. But the loss-of-benefit effect would be blunted because individuals would have an incentive to work so as to pay for additional health care or insurance coverage (in order to receive access and coverage comparable to what they had received before). As a result, the decrease in labor supply would be less, the increase in the equilibrium wage would be less, and the decrease in employment would be less than shown in Figure 2.

Summary

The most likely effects of universal health insurance on low-wage labor markets are higher before-tax wages, higher total labor costs, and lower employment. The analysis of higher-wage labor markets is more complicated, but the results are similar: higher before-tax wages (and higher total labor costs) and lower employment. Our predictions do not appear to be sensitive to the assumptions we have made. Nevertheless, we would emphasize that our conclusions are qualitative, not quantitative, and that the empirical research needed to make quantitative predictions about the effects of universal health insurance on labor markets has not been performed. Filling this gap in the empirical work on labor markets should have a high place on the research agenda.

Mandatory Employer-Provided Health Insurance

In view of its adoption in Hawaii and Massachusetts, mandating has taken on considerable importance as a policy option. Most proposals to require employers to provide health insurance to their workers are coupled with creation of a public program that would sponsor health insurance for anyone who remained uncovered by mandatory employer-provided health insurance. Accordingly, we consider mandating and the public sponsor in tandem.

Mandating is highly controversial, in part because of its potential impact on labor markets. Curiously though, there is broad agreement among labor economists on the general qualitative impact of mandating on labor markets (see Mitchell 1989 for a review). The direct effects of mandating are on low-wage labor markets in which health benefits are not currently provided. There would be two kinds of direct effect. First, to an employer who does not now provide health benefits, the mandating of benefits connotes an increase in the nonwage costs of employing labor [c_i]. This would lead to a reduced demand for labor (in Figure 3, a leftward shift of the demand curve from LD to LD′). Second, the availability of health benefits from low-wage employment—where none had been available before—could lead a greater number of potential low-wage workers to actually offer their services in the low-wage labor market. This implies an increased supply of low-wage labor. (In Figure 3, we show a rightward shift of the supply curve—from LS to LS′—that is relatively small.)[8]

In a labor market where there is no effective minimum wage, the outcome is a reduced wage and a likely decrease in employment. (In Figure 3, the wage falls from w_0 to w_1, and employment falls from L_0 to L_1.)[9] But if an effective wage floor exists in the low-wage labor market, the wage cannot adjust downward. This would occur in the presence of an effective minimum wage, in which case the wage would remain constant, but employment in the low-wage labor market would fall by more than it would if the wage could adjust downward. (In Figure 3, if w_0 is the wage floor, then employment falls from L_0 to L_2. The difference between L_0 and L_2 can be interpreted as the number of workers displaced from this labor market.)

The impact of mandating on higher-wage labor markets would be more subtle, but there are two possible effects. First, mandating would increase the demand for higher-wage workers to the degree that it increased the cost of employing low-wage workers. That is, the higher cost of low-wage labor would induce employers to substitute higher-wage (skilled) workers for low-wage (less-skilled) workers.[10] It follows that the increase in demand for high-wage workers will be greater, the more inflexible are wages in the low-wage labor market (since the total cost of employing low-wage workers rises more when wages cannot adjust downward). We show the impact of mandating on the demand for higher-wage workers by a shift of the demand curve from LD to LD′ in Figure 4. Second, the public sponsor component of mandating could have an impact on the supply of higher-wage labor by providing workers with a relatively low-cost means of obtaining health insurance without being employed. For example, the availability of low-cost public health insurance might increase the likelihood that a worker considering early retirement would actually retire. If so, then the supply of higher-

Figure 3
Effects of Mandatory Employer-Provided Health Insurance
(with a Public Sponsor) on Low-Wage Labor Markets

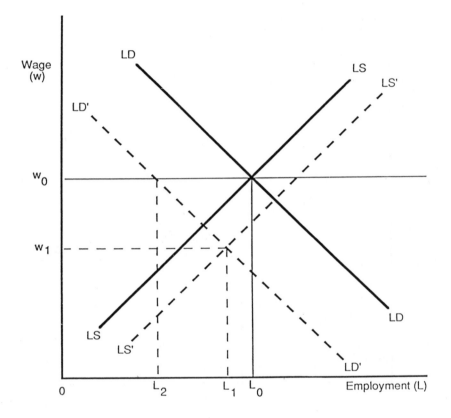

Figure 4
Effects of Mandatory Employer-Provided Health Insurance
(with a Public Sponsor) on Higher-Wage Labor Markets

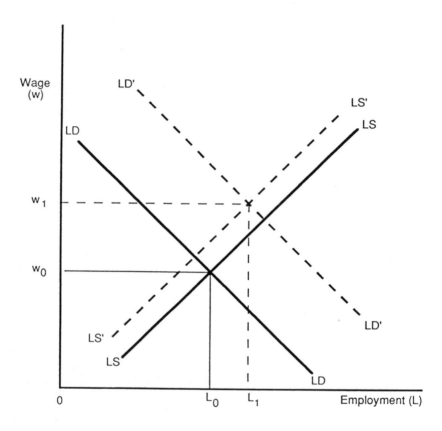

wage workers would fall under mandating with a public sponsor. (See the shift from LD to LD' in Figure 4. We show this as a small shift on the assumption that the labor supply effect of the public sponsor would not be great.) It follows that mandatory employer-provided health insurance (with a public sponsor) would lead to both increased wages and increased employment in higher-wage labor markets (see Figure 4).

Although economists agree on the *qualitative* impacts of mandating, there exists no work that offers *quantitative* estimates of the labor market impacts of mandated health benefits. We urge that high priority be given to obtaining such estimates.

Voluntary Programs to Improve Access to Health Care

Elsewhere in this volume we have explored two so-called voluntary programs to improve access to health care: the Small Employer Health Insurance Pool and Medicaid Buy-In programs for the unemployed and not-in-the-labor-force uninsured. Because a voluntary approach to improving access to health care would involve adoption of both of these programs, it is useful to examine their labor-market effects in tandem.

The Small Employer Health Insurance Pool would reduce the cost of providing health insurance for some employers—mainly small employers of low-wage workers. Specifically, employers who do not now provide health insurance (because their workers are either high-risk or low-productivity) would find the cost of providing health insurance reduced for two reasons. First, creating a pool within which risk could be shared would reduce the premiums needed to provide a given level of health benefits. Second, the policy is designed so that the employer's cost of health insurance is subsidized if the total cost of health benefits exceeds 4 percent of payroll. In effect, the Small Employer Pool would provide a subsidy to employment of low-wage labor by reducing an important nonwage cost of employing low-wage workers (c_i, in terms of our model). Accordingly, the Small Employer Pool would increase demand for low-wage labor (in Figure 5, LD shifts to LD').

Figure 5
Effects of Voluntary Programs
(Small Employer Health-Insurance Pool and Medicaid Buy-In Program)
on Low-Wage Labor Markets

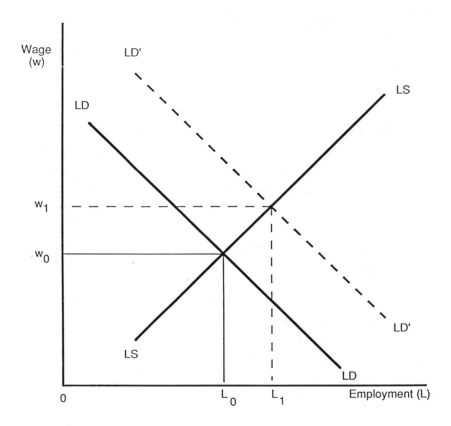

The Small Employer Pool (by itself) would also tend to increase the supply of low-wage labor. The reason is that the existence of health insurance benefits in low-wage jobs that previously offered no benefits would induce more workers to seek work in the low-wage labor market. (In terms of our model, a nonwage characteristic of working in labor market i, n_i, would be improved.)[11]

However, the positive effect of the Small Employer Pool on low-wage labor supply would probably be offset by the Medicaid Buy-In programs that would also be part of a voluntary approach. Since the Medicaid Buy-In programs would allow individuals who are without employment or health insurance to buy a comprehensive package of health benefits (usually at subsidized rates), they would provide an income subsidy for the purchase of health insurance. Such a subsidy implies an improvement in the opportunities available to workers outside of the low-wage labor market (that is, a change in w_j in our model). Accordingly, the Buy-In programs would tend to reduce labor supply to low-wage labor markets. The magnitude of this supply effect would be larger the more generous is the subsidy and the larger is the share of health insurance in low-wage workers' total consumption.

Since the labor supply effects of the Small Employer Pool and the Medicaid Buy-In programs would offset each other, the voluntary programs would have no (or only a very small) effect on labor supply. It follows that the main impact of the voluntary programs on low-wage labor markets would be to increase labor demand, which in turn implies higher wages and increased employment of low-wage workers (see Figure 5).

Whereas the voluntary programs would have a direct impact on low-wage labor markets, their impact on higher-wage labor markets would be indirect. Consider first the impact of the Small Employer Pool on labor supply to higher-wage labor markets. Because the compensation package in low-wage labor markets would improve as a result of the Small Employer Pool (compensation now includes health insurance in addition to wages), fewer workers would offer their labor in higher-wage labor markets. Most likely, this would occur at the margin, as prospective workers leave school and choose jobs and career paths. It follows that the supply of labor to higher-wage labor markets would fall (see the shift from LS to LS' in Figure 6).

Figure 6
Effects of Voluntary Programs
(Small Employer Health-Insurance Pool and Medicaid Buy-In Programs)
on Higher-Wage Labor Markets

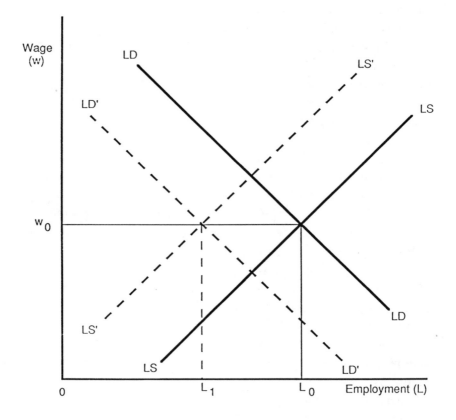

The Small Employer Pool would also influence the demand for higher-wage labor. Because it provides a subsidy to employment of low-wage labor, the Small Employer Pool would induce employers to substitute low-wage for higher-wage workers. As already noted, this implies that the demand for low-wage workers would increase, but it also implies that the demand for higher-wage labor would fall (see the shift from *LD* to *LD'* in Figure 6).

We believe that the Medicaid Buy-In programs would have only a negligible impact on higher-wage labor markets. Accordingly, the impact of the Small Employer Pool on the higher-wage labor market also constitutes the total effect of the voluntary programs on that market. As can be seen in Figure 6, the voluntary programs would tend to reduce employment of higher-wage workers, and would have little if any impact on the wage.

Summary and Conclusions

Because private health insurance coverage is closely tied to employment, policies that are intended to expand the coverage of health insurance can also be expected to have side effects on the labor market. This paper offers both a characterization of the U.S. labor market with an eye to the role of employer-provided health insurance, and a sketch of the theoretical linkages between health policy and the labor market.

The main findings from the statistics we set out in the first section can be summarized as follows.

(1) Roughly 20 percent of all individuals in the United States who worked during 1988 were low-wage workers, earning $5.00 per hour or less (see Table 1). Only 27 percent of these low-wage workers were included in employer-provided group health insurance plans. But 82 percent of these same workers were covered by some form of health insurance. Two points follow from this finding. First, there is far more variation in the degree to which workers are included in employer-provided group health plans than in the degree to which they are covered by health insurance. Second, policies designed to include more workers as the primary insured in employer-provided health plans are less likely

to cover uninsured individuals than are policies that act directly to cover uninsured individuals.

(2) There is much variation from industry to industry in the inclusion of workers in group health plans. Higher-wage industries tend to provide health insurance to a high proportion of their workers, whereas low-wage industries tend to provide health insurance to a relatively low proportion of their workers (see Tables 2 and 3). It follows that policies to expand the inclusion of workers in employer-provided health insurance plans would have an uneven impact, affecting low-wage industries more than others.

We set out a standard model of the labor market that offers predictions about the effects of three policies to improve access to health care. The predictions of the model can be summarized as follows.

(1) Universal health insurance would lead to increased before-tax wages paid to workers, increased total labor costs to employers, and lower employment in both low-wage and higher-wage labor markets. In particular, the belief that universal health insurance would reduce labor costs of employers is not supported by our model.

(2) There is considerable agreement among labor economists regarding the probable effects of mandatory employer-provided health insurance on the low-wage labor market. In the absence of an effective wage floor (or minimum wage), wages would fall and employment would fall somewhat in response to mandating. But in the presence of an effective minimum wage, total costs of employing low-wage labor would rise substantially, and employment of low-wage labor would fall by more than if wages could adjust downward. The increase in total cost of employing low-wage labor would in turn induce employers to substitute higher-wage (skilled) labor for low-wage (less-skilled) labor, and wages and employment in higher-wage labor markets would rise in the long run.

(3) Finally, we considered two voluntary programs to improve access to health care: the Small Employer Health Insurance Pool and Medicaid Buy-In programs for the unemployed and not-in-the-labor-force uninsured. The most important predicted effect of the voluntary programs is an increase in employment, wages, and total compensation in low-wage labor markets. This suggests that the voluntary programs would unambiguously improve the welfare of low-wage workers.

It also seems likely that employment would fall in higher-wage labor markets, although wages would be affected minimally if at all. Since any contraction of higher-wage labor markets would take place over a long period of time, and would result mainly from workers' choices stemming from improved opportunities in the low-wage labor market, we conclude that this contraction would be rather benign from the standpoint of workers' welfare.

NOTES

1. We separate the wage from the other factors in the supply function by a semicolon in order to distinguish factors that result in movements along the supply curve from factors that shift the supply curve.

2. In fact, some low-wage workers do receive health insurance, and some higher-wage workers do not. Our assumptions are made for analytical clarity.

3. See Dickens and Lang (1985) on the appropriateness of dividing the labor market into two sectors.

4. It is also possible that universal health insurance would have an income effect on the supply of low-wage workers. The reason is that some low-wage workers currently use part of their earnings to buy nongroup coverage, but universal insurance would eliminate the need for private purchase of health insurance. As a result, universal health insurance would be like an increase in income to these low-wage workers. The result would be a further reduction of labor supply.

5. Good summaries of the empirical work on labor supply responses to real wage changes include Keeley (1981) and Killingsworth (1983).

6. Two factors could make the tax effect larger, however. First, the effect would be greater if households were pushed into higher tax brackets by the increased taxable earnings that result from severing the link between employment and health insurance (see the discussion of the loss-of-benefit effect below). Second, the wage elasticity of labor supply for higher-wage workers could increase if health insurance were no longer linked to employment. (Currently, benefits are usually provided only to workers who work close to full time, so that higher-wage workers are unlikely to adjust hours as readily as they would if benefits were not tied to full-time employment.)

7. With the exception of work by Atrostic (1982), little is known about the magnitude of labor supply responses to changes in nonwage benefits. Atrostic's work suggests that changes in nonwage benefits have a larger effect on labor supply than do changes in the wage.

8. For two reasons, the effect of mandating (with a public sponsor) on labor-supply would probably be small. First, many potential low-wage workers are (and would be) covered by another family member's employer-provided benefits, as Table 1 demonstrated. Accordingly, many potential participants in the low-wage labor market are insensitive to the provision of health insurance. Second, the creation of a public sponsor to provide health insurance to anyone who remains uninsured would reduce the advantages of obtaining a job that provided health insurance.

9. Note that there is no guarantee that the wage reduction will exactly offset the cost of the newly provided health benefits, as some have contended. Only if the labor supply response were proportional to a labor demand reduction that precisely offsets the costs of mandated benefits would a dollar-for-dollar tradeoff between wages and health insurance occur.

10. In terms of the model, the price (p_j) of an input that can be substituted for higher-wage labor has increased. For evidence on substitution between various groups of labor, see Hamermesh (1986).

11. How many employers would actually participate in the Small Employer Pool is an important topic for further research. There is relatively little work on the reasons for employer participation in government programs, the paper by Ashenfelter (1978) being an important exception.

References

Anderson, John E. "Public Financing Approaches to Improve Access to Health Care." Chapter 7 in this volume.

Ashenfelter, Orley. 1978. "Evaluating the Effects of the Employment Tax Credit." In *Conference Report on Evaluating the 1977 Economic Stimulus Package*, U.S. Department of Labor, Office of the Assistant Secretary for Policy, Evaluation and Research. Washington, DC: Government Printing Office.

Atrostic, B.K. 1982. "The Demand for Leisure and Nonpecuniary Job Characteristics," *American Economic Review* 72 (June): 428-440.

Dickens, William T. and Kevin Lang. 1985. "A Test of the Dual Labor Market Theory," *American Economic Review* 75 (September): 792-805.

Hamermesh, Daniel S. 1986. "The Demand for Labor in the Long Run." In *Handbook of Labor Economics*, eds. Orley Ashenfelter and Richard Layard. Amsterdam: North-Holland.

Hogan, Andrew J. and John H. Goddeeris. "Universal Health Insurance Coverage Through a Single Public Payer." Chapter 3 in this volume.

Hogan, Andrew J. and Stephen A. Woodbury. "Small Employer Health Insurance Pools." Chapter 5.2 in this volume.

Hogan, Andrew J. and Stephen A. Woodbury. "Medicaid Buy-In Programs for Uninsured Children and Non-Working Adults." Chapter 5.3 in this volume.

Goddeeris, John H. "Combining Private Insurance With Public Programs to Achieve Universal Coverage." Chapter 4 in this volume.

Keeley, Michael C. 1981. *Labor Supply and Public Policy*. New York: Academic Press.

Killingsworth, Mark R. 1983. *Labor Supply*. New York: Cambridge University Press.

Mitchell, Olivia S. 1989. "The Effects of Mandating Benefits Packages." In *Investing in People: A Strategy to Address America's Workforce Crisis*, Commission on Workforce Quality and Labor Market Efficiency, U.S. Department of Labor. Washington, DC: Government Printing Office, September.

Woodbury, Stephen A. 1989. "Current Economic Issues in Employee Benefits." In *Investing in People: A Strategy to Address America's Workforce Crisis*, Commission on Workforce Quality and Labor Market Efficiency, U.S. Department of Labor. Washington, DC: Government Printing Office, September.

Woodbury, Stephen A. and Douglas R. Bettinger. In press. "The Decline of Fringe Benefit Coverage in the 1980s." In *Issues in Contemporary Labor Economics and the Implications for Public Policy*, eds. Randall W. Eberts and Erica Groshen. Armonk, NY: M.E. Sharpe.

9
Just Caring
An Experiment in Health Policy Formation
Leonard M. Fleck
Michigan State University

Over the past three years or so, a movement has gradually developed that is described as the "Health Decisions" movement. It refers to statewide, grass roots efforts aimed at stimulating health policy discussions at the community level about many of the more controversial and morally troubling aspects of health policy in the United States. This is an important social and political phenomenon for four reasons. First, these projects have attempted *not* to be just another special interest group in the state. Rather, they have aimed, through public conversation, to identify *common* purposes in health decisions. In analyzing these projects, Bruce Jennings writes that "they have taken pains to avoid polarizing the issues with which they deal. Their objective is to provide a new space for moral and political discourse. This is the space of the democratic forum, where groups that usually confront one another in an adversarial fashion can bracket their differences, at least for a while, and search for common objectives and some common ground. The guiding metaphor of these projects is conversation, not confrontation; and their spirit of advocacy is tempered by one of open and tolerant inquiry" (Jennings 1988, p. 9). This attitude of open and tolerant inquiry should be seen as motivating the project I describe later in this essay.

Second, these projects help to disabuse us of the false belief that our moral concerns and moral conflicts are purely matters of private conscience to be worked out however we wish within that personal inner sanctum. This is especially true when the moral value with which we are concerned is that of justice. If justice exists anywhere, it must exist as a feature of our social policies and practices, not our private consciences. As the philosopher John Rawls observes, "Justice is the first virtue of social institutions, as truth is of systems of thought'' (Rawls 1971, p. 3). Just as truth must be an object of public inquiry through the methods of science, so also justice must be an object of rational public inquiry. The difference is that we have had good models of how science ought to be carried on for the past 400 years. We have had few good models of how public moral inquiry might be done, though the objective of these projects is to create such models.

Third, these projects are important because they reinforce the idea that profoundly moral issues in our public life ought not to be left to political and moral experts, much less managerial, organizational, or economic experts. As Daniel Callahan has noted, there is a strong temptation in our society to treat the problems of health care financing, health care cost containment, and health care rationing as exclusively economic and organizational issues, ignoring entirely the moral dimensions of these issues (Callahan 1990, p. 27). There are reasons why this happens, but they are not good reasons. The issues that need to be addressed are potentially painful and divisive. Health policy options that require us to consider who lives, who dies, and how much we as a society are willing to spend to save or prolong a life are difficult choices. Our social life will be much more pleasant if we can continue to affirm the social illusion that human life is priceless. And, of course, we can get away with just that if we give authority to economic experts to make these choices in think tanks safely sequestered from public view. However, making appropriate decisions in these matters is a moral responsibility that each and every citizen has; and hence, a good democratic society will provide democratic forums and decisionmaking structures that will facilitate the carrying out of that responsibility by its citizens, even though the matters to be discussed are painful and divisive. The fact is that health policy decisions do affect all of us, not just economically, but in profoundly moral ways. *The choices we make with respect to health policy reflect very concretely the extent to which we are a just and caring community in practice.* Symbolic social affirmations of the pricelessness of human life that mask discriminatory rationing decisions privately effected are both dishonest and unjust.

Fourth, if there are limits to what we can and ought to spend on health care as a social good, and if the factors that have precipitated escalating health care costs over the past 20 years are going to continue unabated and even intensified for the foreseeable future, then we will have to accept the conclusion of most health economists that rationing access to health care is inescapable (Fuchs 1974, chap. 1; Thurow 1985, pp. 611-14; Schwartz 1987, pp. 220-24). But, I would argue, we ought not accept the conclusion, advocated by some,[1] that such rationing be effected by institutional mechanisms that are private and invisible, hidden from public scrutiny. I have argued elsewhere that such invisible rationing mechanisms are presumptively unjust.[2] Just rationing policies can be effected publicly. Again, the virtue of the Health Decisions movement is that it has provided us with models of how such public conversations can be productively carried on. It has helped to make these choices visible, painful and tragic though they be.

Though the state projects that have come under the rubric of the Health Decisions movement have had much to recommend them, there has been one major shortcoming. It is that most of these projects have been organized around discrete public forums and workshops that have attempted to address "the" problem of escalating health care costs and equitable access to health care. In point of fact, however, there are at least 20 large problems that can and ought to be distinguished within this policy domain. What virtually everyone who is familiar with this problem domain concedes is that multiple, conflicting social and moral values are at stake, and that tradeoffs need to be made. This last point is something that the larger public will never achieve an adequate appreciation of, so long as their exposure to these issues is in discrete chunks. More sustained and comprehensive public conversations that span months and years are needed to bring about that level of public understanding. What we describe below is a project that represents one model of how that might be done.

In these introductory remarks, I have made what some would regard as debatable assertions which really are in need of intellectual justification, since they ground the practical need for the project I describe. One such proposition is that health care ought to be thought of as a *social* good or public good rather than simply a private consumer good that is properly distributed according to individual ability to pay. This proposition is needed to support the moral claim that there are matters of justice that need to be addressed as part of our choice of health care policies. My second claim is that there are multiple moral problems connected with justice and health policy that need to be addressed and that require, for their resolution, value tradeoffs. During the 1970s, philosophers seemed to think there was really only one moral issue here, namely, whether or not there was something called a right to health care. Anyone familiar with health policy today in its concrete details would see that as a wholly inadequate moral framing of our problem. In the first part of this essay, I attempt to provide a sketch of an intellectual justification for these claims. In the second part, I describe a model for a statewide project that would address, through public conversation, the moral issues that are integral to our health policy choices at both the state and national levels.

Health Care Justice
Who Lives? Who Pays? Who Cares?

The current climate in health care is dominated by multiple demands for health care cost containment. These demands come from both the public and private sectors. The statistics cited most often to portray the problem are the following: In 1990, it is estimated that we in the United States spent about $660 billion on health care, which represented about 12.2 percent of our Gross National Product (GNP). By way of comparison, in 1960 we spent $26 billion on health care, which represented 5.2 percent of GNP then. While the dollar figures are very large, what is most distressing to economists and policymakers is that the fraction of GNP devoted to health care has more than doubled. Worse still, there are few signs in the foreseeable future that escalating health costs will flatten out. Over the past 20 years, health costs have escalated at roughly twice the rate of inflation as measured by the Consumer Price Index, and this has remained true through a major recession during the 1980s and assorted stringent efforts at health care cost containment. Again, by way of comparison, Great Britain spent about 6.4 percent of its GNP on health care in 1989, while Canada spent about 8.7 percent of its GNP. The implication here is that it is possible to spend less on health care;

and, at least in the case of Canada, to have a health care system equal in quality to what we have in the United States (Evans 1986; Evans et al. 1989).

If health care were purchased as a private consumer good, as are all sorts of other consumer goods, then all of the above statistics would have little practical import. For they would simply reflect in aggregated form hundreds of millions of individual consumer decisions to purchase health care rather than something else. However, we do not treat health care as a private good. Rather, since the 1930s we have treated it as a social good, which is purchased primarily through an insurance mechanism, either in the private sector or the public sector. No one doubts that health insurance represents a rational social response to the personal tragedy of serious illness and hospitalization. For the fact is that the occurrence of illness for any individual is mostly unpredictable. Further, in the case of serious illness, there will usually be high costs associated with either cure or relief of the illness, costs that few people would be prepared to meet. It was no coincidence that *effective* health care and health insurance emerged about the same time. What we mean by "effective" health care are interventions that saved lives, prolonged lives, and relieved serious suffering. These are goods to which *all of us* want and need secure access, most especially when we are ill. Health insurance represents one sort of appropriate social response to that need.

While there may be much that individuals can do to forestall the occurrence of many diseases, there is relatively little that individuals can do *as individuals* in response to serious disease once they have been afflicted with that disease. Again, a rational approach to this problem is to devise appropriate *social* responses. Thus, the bulk of medical research and medical education are publicly funded. Physicians have the healing powers they have because a large social investment has been made in them. Moreover, public dollars have built most of the hospitals and paid for most of the technology that makes our health care system effective. As a society, we have even facilitated the purchase of health insurance by exempting that benefit from income and social security taxes, which represented a $48 billion subsidy to the middle class and $48 billion in revenue forgone by the federal government in 1990. It would be very difficult to justify this kind of subsidy, either morally or politically, if what were being publicly subsidized were simply private expenditures by the middle class.

Everything said thus far may be taken as so much stage setting for our primary claim, namely, that there are profound *moral* issues that must be addressed as we make appropriate health policy decisions. For example, in arguing that health care represents a *social good* in our society, what we are implying is that there are important matters of justice pertaining to how this good is distributed, which would not be the case if it were merely another private consumer good. Thus, no one objects to the fact that a unique Picasso painting is sold to the highest bidder, but virtually everyone in our society would be morally outraged if human hearts or livers for transplant purposes were literally auctioned off to the highest bidder. This seems like a solid moral intuition on which there is widespread agreement. But it does not seem to take us very far. If the wealthiest individual with a failing heart or liver has no special moral claim to that organ, who does and who is to decide?

We often think of our society as being meritocratic, which suggests that there are always some individuals who are "more deserving" than others. This makes sense when we are thinking about rewarding individuals for a job well done with a promotion or pay raise. But how would such notions apply when we are distributing transplant organs, which literally will make the difference between life and death. Some may be tempted to suggest that there are individuals who have contributed more to society than others; but certainly this is the sort of claim that could be open to interminable dispute about how we would judge and compare an indefinite variety of incommensurable social contributions. Moreover, many would feel that there was something morally inappropriate and incommensurate in "rewarding" some productive individuals with life while consigning others who were a bit less productive to death.

For those who are inclined to some sort of egalitarian conception of justice, it might seem that because we all have an equal right to life, all who need that organ transplant should at least have an equal chance to get it. This idea has considerable moral appeal. However, the Pittsburgh transplant surgeon Starzl drew significant criticism when he did a liver transplant in 1987 on a 76-year old woman (Koenig 1986). After all, he could have saved more life-years at a lower cost per life-year if a younger patient had received that transplant. This erodes a bit of our confidence in the egalitarian ideal. Then, of course, there are all those patients whose livers or hearts are failing because of their own bad health habits, i.e., an alcoholism problem, or cigarette smoking, or poorly managed stress, etc. Many would feel it is unfair if these individuals have an equal claim to a transplant organ when others have done nothing to bring an organ-destroying illness upon themselves. Most recently, the question was raised of whether individuals who are seropositive for the AIDS virus should have an equal right of access to an organ transplant. It needs to be noted that such individuals will more than likely go on to have the full-blown version of AIDS, from which they will die. However, it could be as long as 10 years before the disease actually manifests itself. In the meantime, this individual has an immediate need for that life-preserving organ transplant.

Nothing said here is meant to suggest there is any easy or obvious answer to these moral problems. There are conflicting intuitions of justice in these cases that pull us (both as individuals and as a society) in various directions. To make matters even more difficult, we need to note that justice is not the only moral value at stake. Many in our society would assert the equal moral importance of affirming the "pricelessness of human life." This value represented "cheap and easy" morality when there was relatively little that medicine could do to prolong human lives afflicted with life-threatening disease. But in an era of rapidly proliferating, expensive, life-prolonging medical technologies, sustaining this value is neither cheap nor easy. And in the real world it often represents a threat to our commitment to justice.

A clear example of how the pricelessness ideal threatens justice is to be found in the Cruzan case in Missouri. Nancy Cruzan was a 25-year old woman in 1983 who was involved in an automobile accident that resulted in her being reduced to a persistent vegetative state for the next seven years. She was sustained in this unconscious state via tube feedings, which her parents asked to have discontinued so that she be allowed to die. Virtually all of the attention of the public and the courts was focused on the issue of whether surrogate decisionmakers have the moral right to choose death for an incompetent patient. But what was ignored was the equally significant moral issue raised by the fact that the State of Missouri was paying $130,000 per year through Medicaid to sustain Nancy Cruzan in that unconscious state, this in keeping with its recently enacted "right-to-life" constitutional amendment. What makes this a significant issue of justice is that the Missouri Medicaid program covers only 40 percent of those below the poverty level, and clearly those other 60 percent could benefit much more from secure access to health care than Nancy Cruzan.[3]

But even if we ignore for a moment these conflicts between justice and the pricelessness ideal, there are substantial difficulties in interpreting what that ideal itself is supposed to mean practically. One way of interpreting what is meant by the pricelessness of human life is to say that a good society will not allow people to die who cannot afford the successful but expensive medical technology that might save and prolong their lives. Our commitment to this belief is most clearly illustrated by the 1972 Medicare amendments that underwrote the cost of dialysis for all those with renal failure. (Prior to those amendments the cost of dialysis, at $30,000 per year in 1968, was a real barrier to access for the vast majority of patients in that condition. Further, there was only one dialysis slot available for every ten patients who needed a slot for survival.) As a result of those Medicare amendments, there are 95,000 people alive today who owe their life to that program. But the cost of that program to Medicare in 1988 was about $2.8 billion. Further, Congress has, of late, strongly resisted any effort to create a similar program that would underwrite the costs of organ transplants, now with a much higher success rate as a result of the introduction of (expensive) immuno-suppressive drugs such as cyclosporine. Major transplant surgery generally carries front-end costs of $100,000 to $150,000 per case. What should we conclude from this lack of political enthusiasm? Do we value human life less now? That is, do we no longer think human life is priceless? If so, should we be subjected to moral criticism? What does justice require in these circumstances so far as our health policy is concerned? Are we treating those in need of organ transplants unfairly, since we refuse to provide public funding for these procedures, especially when we consider that those in need of organ transplants have paid taxes to fund renal dialysis? And what are we to conclude, morally speaking, about the fact that we do fund kidney transplants through the End-Stage Renal Dialysis (ESRD) amendments, but not other organ transplants?

It was announced in October 1987 that the federal government had awarded the University of Utah a $10 million grant over a five-year period to finish the development of a totally implantable artificial heart (TIAH). Unlike the artificial heart that sustained Barney Clark for several months, this heart would not require a 300-pound power source outside the individual. Its power source would be wholly self-contained. On the assumption that this project is successful, how should we respond from a moral perspective? Such a device might be able to prolong the lives of more than a hundred thousand people each year who are in the end stages of heart disease. But the cost of implanting that device in all those people would be more than $12 billion per year, unless we were able to agree upon some set of criteria for rationing access to that device. Here we need to keep in mind that an advantage of the limited supply of natural hearts for transplant purposes is that we cannot escape the need to make rationing decisions. But if we arbitrarily limit the number of artificial heart transplants for political or economic reasons, then we will be saying publicly that there are some lives that *we judge are not worth saving,* even though we have the technology available that could save those lives. That would represent a public repudiation of the widely held belief that human life should be thought of as being priceless. Further, there would be intense public conflict over what represented a truly just distribution of the artificial hearts that were available. At the moment, the choice is still theoretically available to us as to whether or not we ought to fund such technologies. Would we be unjust as a society if we were to choose not to fund that technology?

It would be a mistake to think that the problems we are sketching here pertain primarily to organ transplants. The larger issue pertains to what our societal response ought to be to the occurrence of catastropic illness. As the health economist, Victor Fuchs, points out, health insurance was originally designed to protect all of us from financial ruin by spreading out the risk associated with costly catastrophic illness.

The assumption behind such insurance is that relatively few people would be so afflicted. However, given the continued advances in life-prolonging technology of all sorts, the likelihood is that the vast majority of us will be afflicted with one or more costly episodes of catastrophic illness. That threatens to undermine the whole point of health insurance. The response of insurance companies, as they seek to protect their own interests and those of their clients, has been to increase their vigilance in identifying before the fact individuals who are most likely to suffer such catastrophic illnesses. The best current example would be individuals who are sero-positive for the AIDS virus. Those individuals are then denied insurance, which will mean that they will ultimately be denied needed health care.[4]

The average heterosexual reader should take small comfort in knowing this because, as more tests are developed to identify individuals who are genetically predisposed from birth for certain illnesses, those individuals too will be excluded from insurance pools. It is easy enough to understand the reasoning of insurers in these matters: they will argue that they are not a welfare system, but a mechanism for distributing risk. Still, the net result will be that those who are most in need of health care will most likely be denied access to the health care that they need. This result seems neither just nor humane. But it is clear that this is the direction in which we are moving. Further, where we could once expect that community hospitals would care for these patients as charity care, that is becoming increasingly less true. Hospitals find themselves under intense pressure from purchasers of their services to give discounts, and that effectively eliminates the financial cushion that permitted hospitals in the past to provide charity care.

There are numerous other moral issues that could be fleshed out at this point, but for which space allows only brief allusions. The likelihood of needing a major organ transplant is, I take it, a small probability event for most of my readers. This might undermine my claim that there are issues here that must be addressed by all citizens in our society. However, I would judge that all my readers confidently expect to grow old. The care of the elderly certainly represents a focal point of much moral and health policy attention. The chief reason for this is that the elderly are disproportionately recipients of health resources in our society. Though the elderly represent only 12 percent of the current population in the United States, they are responsible for consuming about 34 percent of all health resources. The twofold emerging problem is that as the post World War II "baby boom" generation ages out, the fraction of this high health care consumption group will grow significantly. Roughly 20 percent of our total population will be elderly in the year 2030, about 62 million people. Further, this problem might be economically manageable if the relative level of health needs per person remained constant into the indefinite future. However, continuing advances in medical technology promise that the health "needs" of this generation will continue to grow dramatically as the elderly live longer and have more chronic health problems for which there will be an increasing number of costly ameliorative interventions.

Given this likely scenario, should we as a society adopt the recommendations of Daniel Callahan and others to identify an age (such as 80) beyond which the elderly would be denied expensive life-prolonging interventions?[5] Or would such a policy be morally objectionable as a form of discrimination comparable to racism and sexism? And what about human growth hormone for the elderly? Recent research suggests that it will improve muscle mass and quality of life for the elderly but at a cost of $13,700 per year per person? (Rudman et al. 1990; Vance 1990). Should Medicare cover those costs? Would it be fair for the public to cover those costs even though there are 37 million Americans without any health insurance at all? And if we are concerned about fair treatment of the elderly and equal moral respect for them, then what are we to conclude about the fact that the Medicare program is a uniform national program, while the benefit package and eligibility levels for Medicaid vary substantially from state to state? Relative to the poor under Medicaid, are the elderly being treated more than fairly, with something more than equal respect? The very asking of this question seems insensitive in the light of great unmet health needs of the elderly in our society, especially their needs for long-term care, home care, and a broad range of social support services. But that only serves to emphasize our larger point: there are real resource limits regarding health care. These limits become painfully evident with every advance in medical technology.

Everything said above may be taken as a very compact sketch of some major problems faced by our health care system today. The conclusions we would wish to draw from this sketch are the following. First, we cannot escape the need to make choices that will involve rationing access to health care, especially expensive life-prolonging forms of health care. The simple fact that economists properly emphasize is that resources are always scarce relative to wants and needs. Second, the problem of rationing is not merely a technical problem to be resolved by economic experts. It is at bottom a moral and political problem, the sort of problem that benefits from the knowledge and advice of experts, but that ultimately must be resolved through the processes of democratic decisionmaking. Third, to improve as much as possible the quality of those democratic decisionmaking processes, it is imperative that there be a broad public conversation of the moral issues that are involved and the policy options that are available to us. Fourth, we are not talking about a single problem that can be easily captured by a single phrase, such as the problem of health care cost containment. This problem spills over and affects a large number of health policy questions, all of which have to be addressed in a comprehensive fashion. What this suggests is the need for public policy conversations among members of the educated public that are sustained and coherent and well informed. Fifth, the most important moral notion that should serve as a focal point for such conversations is the notion of justice. What we need to formulate as a society are just health care policies that will sustain a just health care system. Sixth, we operate with conflicting conceptions of justice in our society, which are often poorly articulated in public forums. We need to improve our articulateness in thinking through our conception of justice.

Seventh, we have no reason to believe there is only one just health policy that somehow all truly rational citizens would agree upon. It is highly improbable that such would be the case. Having conceded that, we do not have to concede that it is impossible to make any moral progress in moving toward more just health policies, for we ought to achieve considerable agreement about those policies or practices in health care that are clearly unjust. If we can accomplish that much through our public conversations, we should regard that as a major achievement.[6]

Just Caring
Health Policy for the 1990s

In the remainder of this essay, I describe a project that we have proposed in Michigan, offering one model of how a socio-moral conversation regarding health care policy might be carried on that is rational
and respectful of our liberal democratic political traditions. It is more
complex than any of the other projects that have been part of the Health
Decisions movement, but I would argue this is what the policy area
itself requires.

Project Goals and Objectives

There have been two projects in the United States that have gotten
a fair amount of national visibility and that provide a useful reference
point for the proper design of this project. Both were *citizen-based* rather
than *expert-based* projects. One was the "Oregon project,"[7] a three-
year project that covered the State of Oregon. It involved over 300 grass
roots community meetings to identify what citizens in general took to
be important moral and public policy issues with respect to health care.
Those meetings took place in almost that number of communities. The
information gathered from those meetings was fed into a citizen's health
parliament, which distilled a number of broad principles regarding the
just distribution of health care resources from those meetings. The problem with this approach is its superficiality at the grass roots level. The
grass roots meetings were more like gripe sessions and less like public
moral conversations in which citizens would have to struggle with making
difficult tradeoffs. That kind of conversation was restricted to the
parliamentary representatives.

The other noteworthy project was from Minnesota. It involved a
distinguished, broadly representative task force of community leaders
and health care providers who sought to articulate principles for the
just distribution of scarce life-saving medical technologies, especially
organ transplants. This project required more in the way of public conversation by project participants, but the range of issues considered was
too restricted, given the real range of tradeoffs that ought to be addressed

within the health care field. Still, both these projects provide us with important guidance. Specifically, they suggest the importance of a project's being *statewide in scope*. That helps to give a project visibility and will help to generate commitment since the project is likely to make a difference in the real world. Next, the project should cover a broad range of issues pertaining to justice and health care policy. There is something that is morally deceptive about taking a piecemeal incrementalist approach to these matters. Finally, the project ought to involve (at least as observers who have an opportunity to question and challenge) as broad a segment of the public as possible.

With the above suggestions in mind, I offer the following as project objectives:

1. To create public forums in which health care professionals and thoughtful citizens can engage in a sustained and systematic discussion of critical moral issues raised by changes in health care technology, health care delivery, health care financing, and health care policy.

2. To raise the overall level of awareness and understanding of these moral issues throughout the state through the judicious use of local newspapers and television, recognizing that only a limited number of people can participate in the face-to-face conversations envisioned under objective 1.

3. To identify and assess from a predominantly moral perspective policy options at the institutional, community, state, and national levels regarding moral issues raised by changes in health care technology, financing, and delivery mechanisms.

4. To identify as clearly and precisely as possible those "considered moral judgments" of justice that the philosopher John Rawls (1971) refers to as the shared starting points for moral conversations that address more controversial moral issues, the assumption being that this is an effective method for reaching some expanded level of agreement with respect to these controversial issues (pp. 19-20, 47-53).

5. To develop a richly nuanced and realistic moral conversation at the state and community levels, one that is both sensitive to the political, economic, and institutional constraints that make "perfect justice" impossible, and that balances what are sometimes several legitimate moral values that conflict with one another.

6. To create institutionalized state and community linkages that will assure the sustaining of this conversation after the project has been completed, in particular, linkages between an informed lay public and institutional providers of health care.

Project Design

Our best judgment is that a project of the sort we have in mind might require three years to complete, probably three years for project planners and two years for project citizen participants. In order to cover a state such as Michigan in some fashion, there should be 15 to 20 project sites, probably located in larger urban areas. (Using Michigan as an example, there might have to be 5 project sites in metropolitan Detroit, given the density of the population. Other sites could include Ann Arbor, Battle Creek, Kalamazoo, Flint, Lansing, Grand Rapids, Saginaw, Midland, Mt. Pleasant, Escanaba, Marquette, Traverse City area, Benton Harbor-St. Joseph area, Petoskey area, Grayling area. For reasons listed below, easy access to a community college, private college, or university is one criterion that should determine choice of sites.)

We envision four stages for a project. The first stage is for detailed project planning. The second stage would be the problem identification/seminar stage. The third stage would be a problem response/activity stage. The fourth stage would involve a summative project conference whose primary objective would be to articulate both a shared vision of what our health policy ought to be and a strategy for getting from here to there. Stages one and four would take place at some central location. Stage one really requires the resources of a large university or a consortium thereof. Stage four requires the visibility of the state capitol. Ideally, stage four would involve a formal engagement with the state legislature and representatives from the executive branch of government. Stages two and three would take place in the various project communities, though there would be substantial centralized coordination and resource provision from the university that served as an administrative home for the project.

Stage One: Planning and Organization

1. *Identify project board and core staff*

The project needs a large Board that will be broadly representative of the different interests and constituencies affected by changes in health policy. Part of the role of the Board is to give visibility and legitimacy to the project. The role of the Board is *not* to "protect interests," but to show that fruitful moral conversation is possible among individuals with diverse interests. That means that the Board itself must be committed to rational "neutral conversation,"[8] as opposed to partisan or ideological conversation. That also means that the capacity for and commitment to critical analysis must be an integral part of that conversation. To help achieve that ideal, it is necessary that there be 10 or so academics from diverse disciplinary backgrounds who will assist the Board (as well as project participants at various sites) in developing and using those critical skills. In addition, some core staff will be needed to coordinate and support project activities at the various project sites. This would include the development and dissemination of materials needed at the various project sites. The importance of this last task should not be underestimated. It takes a lot of creative thinking to design educational materials that will effectively stimulate and focus those community conversations.

2. *Identify broad plan of project activities*

It would be very surprising if the project proposed here is simply adopted by any project Board. We assume that there will be further discussion and revision regarding both the broad design of a project such as this, and the definition of project goals and objectives. Project sites would also have to be identified. It is obviously desirable that population centers be covered, though somewhat rural areas cannot be justifiably ignored since there are important health policy issues unique to that setting. A project such as this needs academic talent at the local level for the reasons cited above, so easy access to such talent ought to be a consideration. Also to be considered are local hospitals who have a Board and/or hospital ethics committee with a serious interest in the goals and objectives of this project. The Goshen project that I directed (which was the small-scale forerunner of this larger sort of project I describe here) was successful because both the Board and the Ethics committee of Goshen General Hospital were intensely committed to the project.[9] An entity that could facilitate access to such institutions in Michigan would be the Medical Ethics Resource Network of Michigan, which is based at Michigan State University, and which links together hospital ethics committees throughout the state. There are at least 15 such networks of hospital ethics committees in other states, which would be seen as an important resource for a project such as this, in part because they will ultimately have responsibility for articulating rationing/resource allocation policies at the institutional level.

3. *Establish a project budget and raise needed funds*

If I were forced to attach some sort of very crude budget figure to the project envisioned here, assuming a total life of three years, I would guess at $35,000 per project site, plus about $300,000 for central planning and administration costs, or about $1 million over a three-year period for a 20-site project. This includes a lot of volunteer effort. But a project of this complexity cannot rely exclusively on volunteer effort. There is simply too much effort and responsibility required at each local site to ensure the success of the project. As for securing funding, it is not unreasonable to pursue state support for this project because it does represent a serious state responsibility; and a project such as this can facilitate legislative decisionmaking. The fact is that legislators are reluctant to undertake any major reforms of health care policy when the policy choices themselves are painful and controversial, and when no more than a small minority supports any particular reform proposal. Other sources of funding include larger foundations in the state and in communities where the project is sited.

4. *Identify local project directors*

A significant commitment of time at the local level would be needed to make this project work. I know that very well from personal experience. Local project directors should be knowledgeable about health care policy and some of the moral issues raised by our policy options. They should have good facilitative and organizational skills, and should feel comfortable working with a highly diverse group of citizens and professionals. They should have some experience with community education. My own biases would incline me toward academics who are successful communicators with a broad professional public, and who are competent in fostering and sustaining the neutral conversation that is necessary for the success of this project.

5. *Identify local planning committees*

These local committees should probably have about a dozen or so members who are broadly representative of key health care constituencies, much like the project Board. This local committee would presumably help with recruiting and identifying individuals who ought to be part of the "core seminar groups" in each community. What we would want are individuals who have a very serious interest in the moral and health policy issues that would be the focus of this project. Working closely with each of these local planning committees would be a mini-academic consortium of three to five individuals who would have pertinent academic backgrounds and who would assist with delivering project seminars/workshops or other such educational efforts.

6. *Hold a planning conference*

The planning conference I refer to here would be for, say, five representatives from each project site. This might really be more of a training conference aimed at making sure that key people at each site understood the goals/objectives of the project, and had some practical direction in recruiting individuals for the "core seminar groups" at each site. Also, strategies for accessing the media should be discussed, so that the project received visibility before a large public and could produce spinoff educational effects in the larger community. Here in Michigan, consortiums of public television stations have worked with one another to develop important statewide programs. Similar arrangements are possible in other states. This project seems ideal for that kind of cooperative effort. Also, in these training sessions there would have to be discussion of mechanisms for stimulating and focusing the conversations that would occur in each of the core seminar groups.

Perhaps the first third of that planning conference ought to be given over to laying out the broad range of problems I alluded to in the first part of this essay for purposes of establishing some shared sense of vision and purpose among participants. The last two-thirds of the program would be given over to exploring various ways in which the project might be implemented at the local level, with special attention given to identifying and resolving potential implementation problems. I envision this as a long one-day conference. That may not be a realistic time frame.

It might also be very desirable to spend a week in the summer training those academics who will have the most direct involvement with the project seminars at each site. Much of that week might be spent modeling, practicing, and testing different ways in which those community seminars might be run. It is critical that there be genuine conversation among seminar participants (as opposed to a series of questions directed to faculty facilitators), and that these conversations be focused and directed.

7. Develop educational resources needed locally

The second stage of the project, what I shall refer to as the community seminar stage, is modeled on the Goshen project that I directed. The central premise of that project was that successful community discussion of issues of justice and health care policy required community conversations that had depth, that were comprehensive, that were well organized, and that were sustained over a period of time. In order to achieve that objective, considerable resources had to be developed in that project, such as newspaper essays, very detailed leader's guides for community seminars, reading materials for each seminar, guides for the work of project task forces, and so on. This required a lot of time and energy, but it certainly resulted in community discussions that were much more focused and productive. If that same effort were required of each project director at the local level, I doubt very many would be interested in attempting the project. Or else project costs would escalate enormously. Consequently, my recommendation is that the educational/publicity resources needed for the project be developed in a centralized way. I can guarantee that this will not produce carbon copy conversations at each site, but will instead facilitate greatly the ease with which such conversations can be initiated.

My suggestion is that for each seminar/workshop there ought to be four to six articles that are required reading for each member of the core seminar group, about 40-50 pages. The sort of articles I have in mind are those that discuss issues of ethics and health policy in professional health care journals, or in publications such as *The Hastings Center Report*. Such articles are generally not excessively academic and opaque.[10] Those articles should be as balanced as possible in terms of reflecting alternative points of view on these policy issues, since there are many reasonable but conflicting points of view on these matters. In the past I also developed leader's guides (four to six typed pages) to accompany each packet of articles. The guides focus attention on specific issues, assist the reader in reading more carefully and critically, and articulate a number of issues that can serve as focal points for discussion in the seminars themselves. The guides also provide cases and exercises for stimulating conversation in the group.

For the project we envision in Michigan, we plan to produce a book-length manuscript organized into 20 chapters that will be coordinated with each of the community seminars that are planned. Each chapter will be a combination of an essay introducing the specific issues that will be the focus of that seminar, and a leader's guide geared to the readings that project participants will be doing for that session. Like the earlier leader's guides, this will also provide specific questions that will give focus and direction to each seminar. The larger objective I have in mind is developing a resource that will have utility as a stimulus for such community conversations elsewhere in the United States.

I also wrote a number of newspaper essays that were published in the Goshen paper just prior to each seminar. These served as a way of involving a larger public in the project. Such essays could also be produced locally for the opinion pages of local papers, depending upon the time and commitment of local academics/participants. This is something that we strongly encourage, because this is a way of drawing these issues to the attention of a public larger than those who can participate in the seminars themselves.

Stage Two: Project Seminars and Workshops

1. *Identify local core seminar groups*

I think there ought to be a "core seminar group" in each community. This could be anywhere from 25 to 50 people who would be invited to be part of the group. About half these people should be connected with health care as providers or administrators or insurors. The other half ought to be broadly representative of the community at large and should themselves be part of the "educated lay public," who understand the importance of reading and are willing to make a commitment to do a fair amount of it. When I say "broadly representative" I mean those groups who are affected in significant ways by health policies. That means both large and small businesses, organized labor, the elderly, the poor, disability groups, and so on.

We would want in this core group people who already have some sort of knowledge base regarding health care policy and the concerns of this project. Members of this core group would commit themselves to attending all of the seminars that would be part of this stage of the project, and they would also commit themselves to participating in whatever activities were part of stage three. They would also commit to doing the reading, since this is the key to having an informed community discussion as opposed to just exchanging prejudices. In the course of organizing this project in Michigan, I have discovered that there is a surprisingly large number of citizens in our society who are significantly involved in health policy groups of one kind or another. These are the sorts of individuals who already have a strong knowledge base in the area, who have the requisite energy and interest, and who would seem to be the group from which seminar participants are most readily recruited. Further, these are the sorts of individuals who will just naturally carry on the project conversation in the larger community long after the formal project has concluded.

Each seminar would last two hours. The first half-hour can be given to a panel presentation or key speaker, just to get things rolling; the rest can be for organized discussion emerging from the readings, the leader guide, or suggested exercises. The public at large should be invited to attend all these sessions, but they are there primarily as observers because, presumably, they will not have invested the time and energy in reading and reflection that members of the seminar group proper will have done. This is not intended to be antidemocratic. Rather, the practical objective is to create a sense of identity and cohesiveness among members of the seminar group proper. My experience shows that this is necessary in order to facilitate the conversational process in the group itself. That is, group members begin to develop a sense of where other seminar members are coming from, which is important for achieving a certain level of psychological comfort necessary for candor. It needs to be kept in mind that the issues to be addressed are both intellectually difficult and emotionally charged.

2. *Seminar topics*

The same topics should be chosen for all the community seminars. Common topics are essential to preserve the statewide nature of this moral and public policy conversation. My recommendation would be that there should be two series of seminars, perhaps 10 weeks for the first set and 8 weeks for the second, with either a winter or summer break, depending upon how they are scheduled. The first series of seminars would serve as an introduction to the major areas of current health policy attention, including the relevant issues of justice, with one seminar focusing on each area. The second series would focus on universal health insurance proposals, or, more generally, proposals aimed at restructuring the way in which we finance health care in America. This latter focus seems to be dictated by emerging policy debates, reflected both in congressional deliberations and in discussions in professional health journals. Though that is a national issue, the issue at the state level that has precipitated that debate is the issue of what ought to be done about the growing number of uninsured in our society, a highly heterogeneous mix whose needs are not readily met by current health financing options.

I am not quite sure how this second series ought to be organized. There are at least eight major credible universal health insurance proposals on the agenda now. Maybe each one of them ought to be a focus of a seminar, the object of which would be to assess each one from the perspective of about a dozen assessment (value) criteria that would have been introduced in the first series of seminars. Of course, one of the options would be that we do nothing at the national level, that each state be left more or less on its own to work out its own policy solutions.

What I imagine as the lead-off seminar at each site would be what I call a "big picture" seminar aimed at giving everyone a sense of the range of health policy issues that must be addressed in public forums and how these issues are connected with one another. That seminar would then be followed by seminars of the sort listed below. Space does not permit a complete listing.

- *Health Care, Justice, and the Elderly.* How might we justifiably set limits on the demands that the elderly make on the health care system, bearing in mind that all of us aspire to be among the elderly some day?

- *Health Care, Justice, and the Poor.* To what extent as a society are we morally obligated to provide for the health care needs of the poor, the uninsured, and the underinsured?

- *Health Care, Justice, and the Terminally Ill, Chronically Ill, and Critically Ill.* How can we justifiably limit the demands that these very needy individuals make on our health care system? Justice may not require doing everything possible, though compassion pushes us in that direction. Still, we are rationally disturbed that we might spend so much and achieve so little in the way of benefit for these individuals. AIDS, of course, fits in under this topic.

- *Justice, Health Care Cost Containment, and the Development and Dissemination of Expensive Life-Prolonging Technologies.* This includes technologies such as organ transplants and artificial hearts.

- *Justice and the Financing of Health Care in America.* Would we have a fairer system for financing health care if we adopted some version of national health insurance, perhaps something along the lines of Canada?

- *Justice and Health Care Cost Containment Approaches.* Assuming that we really must do something to control escalating health care costs, what mix of policies and approaches would be most fair, all things considered?

- *Justice, Health Care, and the Good Physician.* The fact is that 70 percent of all health care dollars are allocated as a result of physician decisions. That effectively makes the physician the gatekeeper to the health care system; and it would imply that he/she ought to be primary rationer of health care sources at the level of the patient. That, however, conflicts with our traditional expectation that physicians will be absolutely loyal to the welfare of their patients.

Stage Three: Critical Value Inquiry

The primary objective of stage three is to acquaint project participants with the broad range of issues we must face more or less simultaneously with respect to making health care policy choices. This will require the making of more systematic, and presumably more thoughtful and more fair, tradeoffs among competing moral and social values. In my mind, the primary objective of stage three is to actually make an effort to work out some set of tradeoffs, and to make explicit the principles and value commitments that govern the choices made. There are really two tasks that need to be undertaken here. The first of these should be the "value inquiry/value tradeoff" task described below. The second should be a working paper in which participants apply the results of their value inquiry to the task of articulating both a state-based and a national policy regarding access to health care. Presumably, this second task should be the natural outcome of the second set of seminars that had focused on the issue of universal access/universal health insurance.

1. *Value inquiry/value tradeoff exercise*

The value exercise I would recommend is based upon something called the "Delphi technique." We start by imagining that as a society we want to commit no more than 12 percent of GNP to health care, which was a little over $660 billion in 1990. Then everyone is individually given a survey form with 70-90 budget items for health care that might be described in some detail. We might ask, for example, whether we should continue to spend $1.5 billion per year to sustain the 10,000 people who are in a persistent vegetative state, just like Nancy Cruzan. Or do we wish to make available 40,000 totally implantable artificial hearts for those under the age of 65 at a cost of $6 billion per year? Or would we be willing to spend $15 billion to make up to 100,000 implants per year available to all who have the relevant medical need regardless of age? Individuals would make their choices among the possibilities up to the specified budget limit. There could easily be $1 trillion worth of choices, which means a large portion of our health wants/ needs would not be funded. To simplify tabulating, we could use a computer score sheet. We would also ask these individuals (the seminar participants) to list the moral principles or other social values they used in making each of their choices. Again, it might be possible to provide a list of 30-50 such "value justification statements" that some-one might choose from. Individuals would be asked to make a copy of their choices for their own records.

All of these surveys would be tabulated at some central site. Par-ticipants would then get two sets of aggregated results. One set would be their local aggregated results, the other would be the statewide results. Seminar participants would then get together to discuss these results among themselves, perhaps for three sessions of two hours each. They could "make a case" for affirming or rejecting whatever the aggregated results were on each item. After this discussion takes place, the same survey is once again filled out by all, and the results are once again aggregated to see what sorts of changes take place as a result of the group interaction and assessment. If people are willing to commit the time, then this second round of aggregated results should be discussed and assessed by the group, after which the survey is completed a third time.

Throughout this exercise it is important to keep in mind two things. First, the objective is not to achieve some sort of agreement on a societal health budget as such. Rather, the objective is to use this budgetary exercise as an effective way to explore the moral and social values in-dividuals believe ought to serve as a basis for making fair and efficient allocations of health care resources. Second, there is nothing morally commendable about one group in society making rationing decisions that will affect the lives and welfare of another group. Hence, it is very important that this exercise be structured in such a way that it is clearly recognized that we are making rationing choices for ourselves and our loved ones. There is a real world circumstance that we ought to be facing up to now, namely, that the post World War II "baby boom" generation is aging out and will make enormous demands on the health care system starting in the years 2010 through 2035. If we, the members of that generation, are unwilling to bear those expenses ourselves, then now we ought to begin making the rationing decisions to which we will bind ourselves in the future.

2. *Critical final paper*

As noted above, each core seminar group should apply the results of the prior inquiry to the task of articulating a policy proposal related to the issue of universal access to health care. Such a paper would reflect the discussions of the group from the second set of seminars, as well as the results of the value inquiry exercise. This is the product that would be brought to the summative conference that would conclude the project.

Stage Four: Summative Conference

This last stage of the project is something that is far from clear in my own mind. It has to be the integrative stage of the project. We might follow the lead of Oregon and Minnesota in this matter and see this summative conference as really a "Health Congress." Each project site would then send some limited number of delegates to this congress. Their task would be to make some specific health policy recommendations that would reflect both the results of the third "Delphi" survey and the papers that had been prepared at each project site. I was recently a participant in a conference that employed a "futures methodology" for defining and integrating the views of the professionals and disciplinary experts who were part of that conference. It struck me that that approach would apply nicely to what we were trying to accomplish here, since this approach involved an explicit integration of values, policy choices and strategies for effecting those policy options. Another possibility is that this "congress" would not just meet on its own. Instead, this would be a sort of joint meeting with the state legislature. Again, a key objective of such a conference would be to engage legislators in the debate rather than to allow them to just listen passively.

From this conference, some sort of public document ought to emerge, though this document would not be a "final report." Rather, it would serve as a starting point for future public moral conversations about the nature of just health care policies and practices. Ultimately, I think it would be desirable if we, as a society, could hammer out something like a "just health care constitution," a practical document that sought to spell out in an explicit and principled way the sort of balances that had to be struck among the many competing values and constraints and considerations that must shape our health care system and health care policy. That requires an even longer and more sustained public conversation, but I believe the sort of project proposed here would make a good start in that direction.

To conclude, a project of this magnitude, properly organized and managed, is likely to have a significant impact in shaping health policy at least at the state level, especially if well managed. It should certainly garner significant media attention. And it should serve as a model for intelligent public policy debate in other states and for other policy areas. One of the things that is assumed is that members of those core seminar groups should be chosen because they have the capacity to educate and influence their constituents or professional peers. What they need to do that effectively are the sorts of resources that would be developed through this project.

NOTES

1. The most vocal defenders of invisible rationing are Guido Calabresi and Philip Bobbitt in their book *Tragic Choices*. The title of their book nicely captures the core of their basic argument, namely, that in matters of health care rationing at the level of social policy, we will always be confronted with tragic choices, choices which will necessarily require that we violate some deep social value. This is because the value conflict is such that to choose one is necessarily to violate the other. Hence, their practical recommendation is that to avoid "exposed choices against life" and "exposed inegalitarianism" (and the social rancor that might be precipitated), these choices ought to be made through social choice mechanisms, such as markets, that will effectively hide the fact that such choices are being made.
2. I have argued against the moral legitimacy of invisible rationing mechanisms in health care in two of my articles (Fleck 1987, 1990a).

3. For a more detailed discussion of this issue, see my article "Pricing Human Life: The Moral Costs of Medical Progress" (1990b). What has emerged more recently is the case of Helga Wanglie in Minneapolis. She is an 87-year-old woman who suffered a very severe heart attack in May of 1990 that resulted in her being reduced to a persistent vegetative state dependent upon a respirator and ICU care. Her husband and two children insist that she herself would have wanted to be sustained in this state indefinitely using all available medical technology. In late 1990, her physicians went to court to ask permission to remove her from the respirator (thereby causing her death) because her care was futile, and there was no medical obligation to provide such care. More noteworthy, however, is that by June of 1991 her care had cost in excess of $1 million. The real issue we need to address here as a society is whether anyone in such circumstances has a just claim on resources of this magnitude. See Miles (1990).

4. For an excellent discussion of these moral issues, see Daniels (1990).

5. See Callahan, *Setting Limits: Medical Goals in an Aging Society* (1987) and Daniels, *Am I My Parents' Keeper? An Essay on Justice Between the Young and the Old* (1988). These two books have sparked an intense debate on the issue of age-rationing. One critical response is Kilner, *Who Lives? Who Dies? Ethical Criteria in Patient Selection* (1990).

6. As noted in the text, I could only present a sketch of the problem of justice as that pertains to health care policy in the United States, and I could only sketch a justification for the moral claims I advanced. The interested reader may find a more detailed analysis in a paper I prepared for the Governor's Task Force on Access to Health Care [Michigan], which has been published as part of the final report of that task force. [See Volume 3, *Background Research Papers*, 109-18.] The paper is titled "Health Care and the Uninsured: Choosing a Just Social Policy." The arguments for the claim that health care policy is a matter of social justice rather than social beneficence may be found in my papers "Just Health Care (I): Is Beneficence Enough?" (1989a) and "Just Health Care (II): Is Equality Too Much?" (1989b).

7. See Crawshaw and others, "Oregon Health Decisions: An Experiment with Informed Community Consent" (1985). A more detailed description is available in a project booklet by Brian Hines, *Oregon and American Health Decisions* (Salem, OR: 1985). More recently, Oregon has garnered considerable media attention for its effort at priority setting and rationing in the state Medicaid program. One of their more controversial tradeoffs would deny organ transplants to Medicaid recipients in exchange for expanding the program to cover 100 percent of the poor in the state as opposed to the current 58 percent. See the article by the physician who is president of the Oregon Senate, John Kitzhaber (1990).

8. This phrase is borrowed from the political philosopher Bruce Ackerman, for whom this is a central practical and philosophic notion in his book, *Social Justice in the Liberal State* (1980).

9. The Goshen project is very well described in a 30-page project booklet available from Goshen General Hospital in Goshen, Indiana. That booklet is titled, *Just Caring: Justice, Health Care and the Good Society*. The project itself was carried out in 1985-87.

10. An excellent example of the sort of essays I have in mind for project seminars are the pieces that David Eddy has been doing in *JAMA* on an occasional basis. They are clear, brief, problem-focused essays that also suggest alternative ways of thinking about issues of health care rationing. These essays nicely integrate the moral, political, economic, and organizational dimensions of these issues. They all appear under the column heading "Clinical Decision Making: From Theory to Practice." The first essay appeared in volume 263 (January 12, 1990). The most recent essay appeared in volume 265 (May 8, 1991). There have been 13 essays so far.

References

Ackerman, Bruce. 1980. *Social Justice in the Liberal State.* New Haven: Yale University Press.

Calabresi, Guido and Philip Bobbitt. 1978. *Tragic Choices.* New York: Norton.

Callahan, Daniel. 1990. *What Kind of Life: The Limits of Medical Progress.* New York: Simon & Schuster.

_____. 1987. *Setting Limits: Medical Goals in an Aging Society.* New York: Simon & Schuster.

Crawshaw, Ralph et al. 1985. "Oregon Health Decisions: An Experiment with Informed Community Consent," *Journal of the American Medical Association* 254 (December 13): 3213-16.

Daniels, Norman. 1990. "Insurability and the HIV Epidemic: Ethical Issues in Underwriting," *Milbank Quarterly* 68: 497-525.

_____. 1988. *Am I My Parents' Keeper? An Essay on Justice Between the Young and the Old.* Oxford: Oxford University Press.

Evans, Robert. 1986. "Finding the Levers, Finding the Courage: Lessons from Cost Containment in North America," *Journal of Health Politics, Policy and Law* 11: 585-615.

Evans, Robert et al. 1989. "Controlling Health Expenditures: The Canadian Reality," *New England Journal of Medicine* 320 (March 2): 571-77.

Fleck, Leonard M. 1987. "DRGs: Justice and the Invisible Rationing of Health Care Resources," *Journal of Medicine and Philosophy* 12 (May): 165-97.

_____. 1989a. "Just Health Care (I): Is Beneficence Enough?" *Theoretical Medicine* 10 (March): 167-82.

_____. 1989b. "Just Health Care (II): Is Equality Too Much?" *Theoretical Medicine* 10 (October): 301-10.

_____. 1990a. "Justice, HMOs, and the Invisible Rationing of Health Care Resources," *Bioethics* 4 (April): 97-120.

_____. 1990b. "Pricing Human Life: The Moral Costs of Medical Progress," *Centennial Review* 4 (Spring): 227-53.

Fuchs, Victor. 1974. *Who Shall Live? Health, Economics, and Social Choice.* New York: Basic Books.

Jennings, Bruce. 1988. "A Grassroots Movement in Bioethics—Community Health Decisions," *The Hastings Center Report* 18 (June/July).

Kilner, John. 1990. *Who Lives? Who Dies? Ethical Criteria in Patient Selection.* New Haven: Yale University Press.

Kitzhaber, John. 1990. "Rationing Health Care: The Oregon Model." In *The Center Report* 2 (Spring). Denver: Center for Public Policy and Contemporary Issues, University of Denver.

Koenig, Richard. 1986. "As Liver Transplants Grow More Common, Ethical Issues Multiply," *Wall Street Journal* (October 14): 1, 32.

Miles, Steven. 1990. "Why A Hospital Seeks to Discontinue Care Against Family Wishes," *Law, Medicine, and Health Care* 18 (Winter): 424-25.

Rawls, John. 1971. *A Theory of Justice.* Cambridge: Harvard University Press.

Rudman, D., et al. 1990. "Effects of Human Growth Hormone in Men Over 60 Years Old," *New England Journal of Medicine* 323 (July 5): 1-5.

Schwartz, William. 1987. "The Inevitable Failure of Cost Containment Strategies," *Journal of the American Medical Association* 257 (January 9).

Thurow, Lester. 1985. "Medicine Versus Economics," *New England Journal of Medicine* 313 (September 5).

Vance, M.L. 1990. "Growth Hormone for the Elderly?" *New England Journal of Medicine* 323 (July 5): 52-54.

INDEX